A PROPER WEIGHT LOSS PROGRAM AND IMPROVING HEALTH

A PROPER WEIGHT LOSS PROGRAM AND IMPROVING HEALTH

Using the Latest Science and Technology Concepts

KOUROSH NAZIRI (CYRUS)

Ordering Information:
You may search this book in Amazon, Barnes & Nobles and other online retailers by searching using the ISBN below.

Copies of this book may also be obtained by inquiring at
www.cyrusn21century.com with discount.

ISBN (Paperback): 978-1-952062-76-6
ISBN (Hardcover): 978-1-952062-83-4

[City]
Book Review
SAN FRANCISCO | MANHATTAN | SEATTLE
PORTLAND | KIDS' BOOKBUZZ

A Proper Weight Loss Program And Improving Health
By Kourosh Naziri (Cyrus)

Star Rating: 5/5

A Proper Weight Loss Program and Improving Health by Kourosh Naziri (Cyrus) is an enjoyable read overflowing with valuable bits of information. The author has crafted a well-organized, approachable book to support and guide readers through their individual health quest. This is not a book written by a medical professional laden with clinical jargon that will overwhelm and discourage readers. Every section provides thoughtful recommendations related to diet, exercise, and overall wellbeing to improve an individual's quality of life. With that said, Naziri (Cyrus) encourages readers from beginning to end to discuss any health-related changes or ideas that come to mind prior to introduction with a healthcare professional. The author is not a doctor or scientist in the medical field, he has simply acquired invaluable information that he willingly shares with his readers. His suggestions are not easy but they are simple. Drink more water. Practice consistency in your diet and exercise. Listen to your body. Seek the guidance of specialists and advocate for yourself. Through these actions, a number of ongoing and future health concerns will be eliminated. He breaks these principles down between two sections, the main part of the book and the annexes. The main part of the book contains information that is beneficial across age groups and capabilities. This section covers principles to live by that range from regular exercise to dietary standards for harmful elements typically ingested in high amounts, such as fat, sugar, and salt. Naziri (Cyrus) encourages readers to focus on enjoying the proper amount of all food groups, particularly proteins and fiber-rich vegetables that tell your body what to expel, what to consume, and how best to operate. The annexes expand on these subjects with additional detail and provide demographic-specific recommendations, related to gender, age, and pre-existing medical conditions. Together these pieces create a comprehensive program that will aid in weight loss and a person's overall improvement of health. Kourosh Naziri (Cyrus) has assembled an effective, informative resource that readers will find accessible, helpful, and engaging. The information is far from overwhelming and builds on our common sense knowledge. The author describes the book as "easy reading for ages of nine to ninety-nine," which demonstrates the approachable nature of the work. With that said, the author urges young readers to enjoy the book under the direct guidance of a parent or teacher who can offer additional instruction and explanation. *A Proper Weight Loss Program and Improving Health* stands as an exceptional example of health and wellness information presented in a simple, user-friendly manner.

-Reviewed by Jessica Tingling || San Francisco

[City]
Book Review

SAN FRANCISCO | MANHATTAN | SEATTLE
PORTLAND | KIDS' BOOKBUZZ

Depending on your level of enthusiasm towards losing weight and learning ways to excise better. Reading Proper Weight Loss Program and Improving Health might be for you. At least you'll be reading something that might motivate you to get started.

The book has the two section. The first is about diet and exercise. while the second contains annexes that cover questions related to health. The author makes it clear in the introduction and preface that his purpose is to create a book that is easily understood and accessible for people aged 9-99 years old.

Kourosh Naziri (Cyrus) appears to mean well with the information he has provided. He claims that he has personally tested many of the pieces of advice offered, consulted a doctor, attended seminars, read articles, ad learned about dangers related to being overweight and unhealthy as well as how certain foods can play a role.

Being a reader who also places a value on healthy(ish) eating and exercising to improving one's overall health, I appreciate his attempt to make the topic better known.

I don't believe that the author will do much harm with this book, though, and at least you'll read about some truths like how sugar in excess is harmful and how exercise is good.

-Reviewed by Rachel Dehning

Seattle, Portland Book Review

A Proper Weight Loss Program And Improving Health
By Kourosh Naziri (Cyrus)

A Proper Weight Loss Program and Improving Health is designed to help regular people aged 9-99 to lose weight and thus improve their health.

The book is divided into two sections. Section One sets out the principles that the author believes will lead to a healthier life and more active lifestyle. These principles include the importance of eating the same amount at the same time each day, exercising more after eating more, and replacing high-sugar and high-fat foods with alternative options. Some of the principles are accompanied by examples from the author's life, others by practical exercises that readers could try for themselves. Section Two contains a number of annexes, some targeted toward certain sections of the population (those aged 50 and above; children; men and women), some that reiterate information from the main body of the book, and others that briefly introduce new concepts, such as the utility of drinking tea and coffee.

Some of the information provided in the book is well-known, common-sense stuff.

Being very much based on the author's personal philosophy regarding health, *A Proper Weight Loss Program and Improving Health* contains a lot more opinions than facts. The author regularly mentions talking to doctors about his ideas and researching health- related matters in books.

INTRODUCTION

This book is a result of over 30 years of research, studying, attending seminars, interviews with a lot of doctors and health professionals, and watching videos, etc. I have had a fascination with medical science, although my formal education is on electronics. I am a former electronics lecturer at Northern Virginia community college, a former data network specialist at the World Bank. I was thinking that maybe my fascination comes from my family. It might be interesting to note that, in my extended family we have over 100 medical doctors, dentists, and all other health professionals.

In this book, I have tried to keep an eye on the 21st century and its issues. Most of us now, use modern transportation, TV, computers, cell phones, and other technology. This does not require any physical activity. But in the old days, we used more physical activity in our jobs and our lives. For transportation, we used riding on horseback or walking, etc. Our tastes have changed too. People now eat fattier, saltier and sweeter foods that might create health complications.

I have discussed some principles about diet and exercise that I got from experts in nutrition and health sciences. Some other principles are from my deduction and by subsequent experiment. Once you apply these principles you'll realize how easy it is to follow the diet and exercise plan that I have brought up. A lot of people find these principles to make the diet and exercise very joyful and rewarding.

I have included some of my experiences, in this book. I have personally lost close to 80 pounds. Also, I have improved my health beyond my expectations. For example, I noticed, that my pulse rate has been reduced, suffice it to say that, I found diet and exercise very rewarding, in terms of weight loss and improving health.

I have tried very hard to make this book easy reading and simple to understand. I intended to make it understandable to people of ages 9 to 99. Kids and young women and men who are under maturity age might find the annex one very interesting. I specifically I am referring to a question and answer. The question is can people make themselves taller by organic means?. If you're interested in this subject, please see annex one. I have tried to leave the medical jargon out of the book. I like to think of this book as a book of weight loss and improving health. I have concluded through my studies and my experience, that weight loss and improving health go hand-in-hand. It is my opinion that obesity and being overweight are the root causes of a lot of undesired illnesses. Some of these illnesses could lead to very harmful, and even health threatening illnesses. For example, obesity, and being overweight could cause diabetes, heart attack, and stroke, according to the articles that I've read and doctor interviews. One of the very main ideas of this book is to prevent it. A doctor told me that "sometimes I have seen health improvement to the point of taking some of the abnormalities in your blood to the normal level". It is as important to lose weight and -improve health, by keeping proper diet and exercise. We will discuss all of these subjects in the book. This book is intended for ages 9 to 99. Meaning it is easy reading. But especially children of up to say 15 years old, should be under some kind of supervision. By supervision, I mean, in the first place the parents. Secondly, I know at gyms, or in high schools or schools, there are gym teachers that can guide you for better performing the exercises, to say the least. Furthermore, it's worth it, to invest in yourself or your child to take them to the specialist applicable to what he or she is about to do. By specialist, I mean something like a cardio specialist for determining the person's optimal[1] heart rate that we will discuss in this book how important this rate is. This is the rate that keeps you healthy, lose weight[1] and more. The exercises especially the back exercises you might want to consult with a chiropractor or orthopedic, to get the best answer. I think to put yourself in the hands of a specialist who is trained and educated and experienced, is a very wise idea.

I want to mention that this book is about improving your health and losing weight. I had no intention of this book to be for bodybuilding or people who like to exercise with heavy weights etc.

1: see optimum heart rate in the book "Fit or fat" By Dr Covert Bailey

PREFACE

For children that are under age, especially under 15 years old, parental guidance is strongly recommended for this book, for exercises and using the small electronic heart rate monitor.

This book is intended, to be easy reading for ages of 9 to 99. Although this book intended mostly for adults, who want to have better health, and lose weight. This book could be useful for all ages. I specially have included an appendix, especially for very young people. Under the parent's discretion, these very young readers could read and apply the annex one.

This book is comprised of two sections. Section 1 is the main body of the book. It shows you how to diet and exercise. Section 2 is called annex chapters. It is used for both reading and reference. The best way is, to read section 1, and then read the categories that are appropriate for you in annexes. For example, some of the chapters in section 2 are for very young readers, or some other, could be for people age 50 and older, etc. Diet and exercise should be joyful for you. It is emphasized that in my opinion if you are pushing yourself too hard, or straining yourself through diet or exercise that means you are doing something wrong. I have also shown a way for people who like to eat a lot. I will answer such questions as: is there a diet that helps you eat all you can eat. There are exercises that make you lose weight at the same time are joyful to you.

Section 1 contains some principles that although they might seem simple enough, never the less they are very effective. These principles are obtained from my interviews with health professionals and doctors, also by my deduction -and- practical experience. In my opinion fat is the most dangerous substance in the body. There is a vast pool of fat across the body, underneath the surface of the body, i.e. mostly under skin and tissues. This is a danger that could kill a lot of people. In my opinion, too much fat content in the body is the mother cause of many illnesses that you don't want. To name a few, I can say, cholesterol, which leads to heart attack, and/ or stroke. Please read the following pages for more information. For example, I believe even the blood sugar level is influenced by the amount of fat in your body. Based on my interviews with experienced and knowledgeable doctors I know for fact that, pre-diabetes, for some people, can be cured by weight loss, proper exercise, and diet. Also, the amount of cholesterol is influenced by the amount of fat content in your body. Many other examples are brought up in the main body of the book.

Section 2 contains independent chapters that are for a special category of people. For example, there is a chapter for younger people or another chapter is for people who have pre-diabetes. For example, Kids and young women and men who are under maturity age might find annex one very interesting. I specifically am referring to a question and answer that discusses a subject, i.e. getting taller. Can people make themselves taller by **organic means** without hormones and all of these other funny substances and drugs? If you're interested in this subject, please see that annex.

The purpose of these chapters is, not only, to add to the contents of the first section, but also serve as a reference and quick reading for people of that category. For example, you might want to know the principles that apply to the body, not storing fat and consuming the fat for energy and so forth. I recommend to the readers to read maybe even glance at least the chapters that might not apply to you right now, for the prevention of certain health problems in the future.

SECTION ONE

THE MAIN PART OF THE BOOK

CHAPTER ONE

TELL YOUR BODY NOT TO STORE FAT, AND CONSUME IT TOO

As mentioned earlier in the pre-face, my book is based on some principles. The first principle is how to tell your body not to store fat and consume it. You should have a very good diet and exercise plan for yourself. We will discuss a lot of these strategies in the following pages.

First principle of "tell your body not to store fat and consume it too."

Use the biological clock

I have tested and re-tested all of these following matters that I am about to bring, on the subject of "tell your body not to store fat and calorie it too".

There is some kind of logic and rhyme-and-reason for everything that our body does. The only brain in the body is in the head. But how do the different parts of the body or organs perform their duties? Or specifically for the discussions of this book, how does your body know how much fat to store or whether to consume the fat or store it. The amount of food or the kind of food are very decisive factors. Usually, if you eat more than your body needs, a lot of it has to be turned into fat, and hence body weight will go up. As another example, if you eat butter with your bread or any kind of fatty substance in other foods as add on, obviously the fat in the butter is so easy[1] to turn into body fat. Or other examples[1], fried food, or any food that has any kind of fat in it, can easily turn into body fat and body fat means gaining weight. The next category[1] after fat is carbohydrates like bread, rice, potatoes, all kind of macaroni or starchy foods. This category is better in terms of not gaining weight than the fat category. But the worst of carbohydrates is sugar. We will touch this subject a little bit here. The food that muscles or body parts can use is some kind of sugar. So by eating sugar, you make the work easy for your body. The idea is to make it as hard[1] as possible for the body to turn the food into sugar. If you have too much sugar in the body, then the excess sugar will turn into fat. Perhaps the best category[1] in terms of not gaining weight amongst the three kinds of nutritious categories is the protein foods. By protein, I mean fish, chicken, veal, turkey, beans, and more. Now this category is harder to turn into the necessary food for the body parts i.e., sugar. There is another group, the green vegetables. Generally, the green vegetable group, or cauliflower etc. don't increase your body weight. This group of foods, as a general rule, have a lot of fiber in them. Fiber helps your digestion, and it's not easy to turn to sugar or fat. So although the green vegetable group as a general rule are not nutritious, however, it's a

1: Fit or Fat by Dr Covert bailey

1

very good supplement to the nutrition that you need. This way your digestion would be helped by this fiber and fibers are good fillers i.e. they fill your stomach and reduce your hunger. More advantages of the fiber group will be discussed later. However, there are other factors that people might not pay attention to. There are some principles in the next few pages that will illustrate these points. On the first principle, you will see that for example by changing your eating schedule you are doing yourself a favor. And the favor I'm talking about is by changing or adjusting your eating habits. Then you would be telling your body not to store fat and consume it for energy better than the others who don't observe this principle.

The First principle is based on the biological clock in our body that I have read about. In simple terms the body expects things to happen regularly. For example, your body needs food during breakfast at a certain time every day say at 8 am. That is why, your body secrets acid, so that you feel hungry. Here's my fine point, the best way to make your body to understand that, not to store fat but also consume it, is in this example to eat breakfast every day at 8 am. The same way for lunch and dinner. That means you eat lunch at a certain time every day no matter if it is a weekday or a weekend, holiday or whatever. So eat each meal every day at the same time. Perhaps it can be said that, if you don't provide the food at exactly 8 o'clock in that example above then your body thinks that it's better to save some Fat just in case, the food is not presented to the body at 8 o'clock that we discussed. So in this example, if the food is given to the body at exactly 8 am., then the body is relaxed in terms of knowing that the food is coming on time in the same amount and it will not go into fat saving mode. The same principle applies to exercise. That means your body expects to have exercised the same amount that you do every day and exactly at the same time. Now a question: do you have to eat at the same time looking at your watch by even seconds and minutes? The answer is that there is a Grace period. Your body has a tolerance of say half an hour or maybe one hour according to my own experience. So for example, if on an occasion you are late for lunch as much as one hour you're still OK or if you eat one hour earlier at the maximum, still alright. For your information, this principle is deducted by me and I have not read it anywhere. Furthermore, I have tested and retested these facts mentioned above many times.

This first principle, in my opinion, can help to reduce heartburn and other digestion problems. Aside from health complications of not eating on time, the point I was trying to make in the previous paragraphs, was that eating smart is always better than any other way. This way by eating smart you are clearly on your way to lose fat i.e. lose weight and also improve your health.

In a nutshell, this principle says that, eat your meals and snacks, at the same time every day, and the same amount every day. By the same token exercise the same amount every day, and also the same time every day.

Second principle of **"TELL YOUR BODY NOT TO STORE FAT, AND CONSUME IT TOO."**

The roller coaster

A question, have you heard of people, who starve themselves for some time or skip a meal? Or have you seen people who believe that some kind of rotational eating is a good idea? An intelligent person will immediately think of the first principle mentioned above, this principle states that you should eat the same amount of food every day at the same time. The second principle is called the roller coaster principle. Do not ride on a weight-loss roller coaster. What that means is, some people eat so much one day, and yet another day or following days go on severe diet or starvation or perhaps skip a meal. The same rule applies to exercise. Too much one day, and less or no exercise the following days. These roller coaster riders think that by doing this they are doing themselves a favor. They are not. They are putting themselves on a bad roller coaster ride, which makes your body to store more fat, and gain more weight. The first day that they eat so much the body goes into fat saving mode. Then the following meals, the person goes on a severe diet again the body goes into a deeper fat saving mode. The body at this stage in its mind thinks that since the food supplies are cut off , it better go into severe mode of fat saving. That's how you start gaining weight. The more you play with the amount of food you eat, and as a result put the amount of food on a roller coaster the more fat you are going to gain, and hence your body weight is going to go up. The same rule applies to exercise, which means exercise same amount at the same time every day.

Third principle of "Tell your body not to store fat and calories too."

Breaking diet and exercise

I know on occasions, people have to go out with their friends for example, or at family gatherings, they can't always keep their diets. So I have a solution for you. When you go out and have to eat a lot of food, or foods that are not diet, then in the next available time preferably within few to several hours you need to exercise so that the foods you had the previously, for example, will be calorized. For an average person, I recommend say one hour of rigorous exercise like jogging or bike riding or a stationary bike. But I must remind you that if you have any health complications that prevent you from jogging or rigorous exercises then you put that matter up with your doctor. As always, I say that you do exactly what the doctor has ordered.

The fourth principle of " TELLING YOUR BODY NOT TO STORE FAT AND CONSUME IT TOO"

Activate and reactivate your muscles

Activate, reactivate and develop as many muscles that you usually don't use in exercises, including walking. I have come up with a new way of exercising that I have personally tested, I know it could be a very effective way of exercise and losing weight. You are using all of the muscle groups that you can think of, that can be used during exercise. By doing so, you will develop newer and stronger muscles in those newly activated muscles. The more muscle you have the more fat you consume, and less fat that you store in the body. Obviously, during the whole exercise, you must keep a straight posture. That means no arches in the back. The back is comprised of the lower back, middle back, and upper back. Try to put all of your back into exercise, your buttocks, front and back leg muscles, calf muscle and your stomach too. To do this try to put pressure on the muscles mentioned. You should feel that you are pressuring the muscles. Your back has 5 parts in my opinion, but I usually have seen 3 parts according to the sources that I have investigated. I have found out that the middle back actually has 3 parts i.e. lower middle, middle and upper-middle back. Word of caution is that your heart rate goes up, by using more muscles, I would observe the heart rate monitor every 5 seconds better yet stare at your heart monitor during exercise. See chapter 5 for a very small electronic device called heart rate monitor. This is seriously important.

Fifth principle of "telling your body not to store fat, and consume it too"

Replace sugar and fat with other tasty foods

Cut down sugar and fatty substances from your diet. I like to recommend something for people who love sugary things. Anytime you have an urge for sugar, eat a piece of, banana or sweet fruits. I like to mention that number one fruits have a lot of fiber in them. Secondly, the sugar in fruits is a lot easier to consume than regular sugar due to the fiber contents. Also, people who love to eat the so-called, greasy foods, perhaps you can compensate for the taste with something like spices or honey or other things. I have mentioned in the following pages, some healthy and delicious munchies. For example, use nuts[1] or fruits, etc. it is worth mentioning that even nuts have fat in them even fruits have sugar in them. However, as long as you keep moderation you should be alright.

The best substance in terms of being hard to turn into fat is fiber[1]. The next best group[1] is the protein group; I guess you call it in layman terms the meat group. After[1] that are the carbohydrates or starchy foods. And finally the worst i.e. the bottom of the list is the fat[1] itself. A lot of the food that we eat has[1] something from one category and some other thing from another category. For example, beans have protein and fiber in them.

1: Fit or Fat book by Dr Covert Bailey

CHAPTER TWO

Principles of "tell your body not to store sugar in the blood and consume it too."

I call Sugar the poison powder. This powder is used in cakes, snacks, cookies, etc. From what I understand, it's very popular. Meaning a lot of people use it every day. For example, in a 12 ounce can of soda, on average, you will find 8 teaspoons of sugar. Sugar is easily turned into fat. Sugar is a carbohydrate. It is top of the list of this group as being the worst in terms of turning into fat so easily. From what I have heard sugar is one of the major causes of diabetes and pre-diabetes. Sugar creates a substance in the blood called triglycerides. Triglycerides from what I was told by a doctor, for some people, cause clotting of the arteries, especially people with pre-diabetes or diabetes. And we all know how dangerous that is. If clotting of the heart arteries happens, there is a great chance of heart attack. I don't know for fact, but I presume that clotting of the artery that is going to the brain might cause a stroke.

In this chapter, we will discuss a few principles to perhaps neutralize, and consume some of the sugar in the blood.

First Principle of "tell your body not to store sugar in the blood and consume it too."

Principle of fiber group.

Fibers are found abundantly in green vegetables, and more such as cauliflower and fruits. Of course, fruits have sugar in them as a general rule. So if you only want close to pure fiber, eat more green vegetables. However, fruits are not bad either. You will see a discussion of fruits and their fiber in the following principles. I attended a seminar that the speaker was talking about blood sugar and the effect of fibers on blood sugar. Fibers will neutralize the sugar in the blood. That means the more fiber you eat, the more sugar you're going to neutralize in your body. Once again I want to emphasize that, if you have any health conditions, the author of this book will not accept any responsibility. The responsibility is between you and your doctor. Simply because the doctor knows what to tell you and what to prescribe and what not to prescribe. For example, if you have any kind of diabetes or prediabetes or any allergies, I would recommend that you talk with your doctor.

Principle of sugar substitutes

The best sugar substitutes that I know of are the ones that are found in fruits, and Honey. From what I understand from a doctor, these kinds of sugars are consumed better and faster, due to fiber contents and therefore they won't stay in the blood. Moderation is an important factor. Meaning it's wrong to assume that, if you sit and eat fruits and honey all day you won't gain weight or your blood sugar won't go up. What I'm saying is though that, if you substitute sugar with fruits or honey, and if you have moderation in mind then you should be alright. Then again responsibility is not mine, is between you and your doctor, especially if you have any kind of health condition. For example, if you have an excess of triglycerides or too much sugar in your blood don't hesitate to get an appointment with your doctor before you do anything. So if you have an urge for eating something sweet, why not a piece of fruit or use honey to sweeten the nuts you're eating or the food you're eating, also the sauces that you use as an add on to your food. Furthermore, the sugar found in fruits and honey by my own experience proved a point to me. The creation of triglycerides, in the blood. That means from my own experience and blood tests that I have taken, it is proven to me that these kinds of sugars that I discussed i.e. sugars in honey or fruits, will not create as much triglycerides in the blood. Again fibers might be the reason.

Third principle of "tell your body not to store sugar in the blood and consume it too."

Exercise

A doctor also told me that, people who exercise, as a general rule, will have better stamina. For example, he continued, if you are one of the people who catch cold and other diseases so easily, perhaps the best solution for you is to exercise to raise your stamina. It is also known that perhaps exercise is the secret of youth. Also, it is a known fact that, exercise especially, if you sweat, will get rid of a lot of bad chemicals from your body. People who exercise as a general rule are more optimistic, more energetic, and feel better about themselves.

Exercise is a very important factor to consume sugar and keep it away from the blood. Of course, the more rigorous exercises perhaps are more effective in terms of sugar consumption. I was told by an expert who was lecturing on blood sugar and its complications, that heavy exercises such as weight lifting are also very effective for this purpose.

CHAPTER THREE

little salt is very essential for the body, and the lack of salt could make you sick. A doctor told me, that too much abstinence of salt, drops your blood pressure to dangerous levels. Salt used, as I can remember from my college courses, is used for reconstruction or regeneration of body cells. So as you see, it is very necessary to take some amount of salt with your food. Also as I remember from one of my courses in college the amount of salt that body can use constructively is about one small pinch of salt per day. However, the situation is more complicated than that. Every food that you buy from restaurants or coffee shops etc. already has salt in it. If you use ketchup or other condiments, or cheeses, etc., they also have some salt in them. So let's say for an average person a small pinch of salt is more than enough per day. Furthermore, salt is known for the fact that it raises blood pressure. So people who have high blood pressure could start by cutting down the salt intake drastically. Like I have personally experienced, you can run a test on your own. If you have a blood pressure check device, test your blood pressure, before and after, cutting down salt for say a few days.

Salt has another effect on the body. It makes your body to hold more water. So the more salt you take the more water you're going to hold in your body. As a result, your weight will go up, due to the water gain in your body. However, that's not the only complication. As your weight goes up your body has to reserve more fat. As a result of extra salt, your bodyweight will go up again and again.

The second subject is fat. It is a simple fact that we don't want too much fat in our body. There are many shapes and forms of fat[1] as food. For example, it could be butter, cooking oil, any kind of fried food. When I say fried, it could be deep-fried also. Naturally, a smart person will avoid fat. The fat, to make it in simple language, as an intake, can easily turn into body fat without much effort[1]. Again fatty foods are very delicious. A lot of people, to make their food delicious, they add fat and salt to the food. Both fat and salt are among some of the most damaging substances to the human body.

Fat causes an increase in cholesterol in the blood. From what I have read in the articles cholesterol is in the fat or oil category or families. I also read, that cholesterol makes the arteries and veins more flexible, and helps the flow of blood in them if I remember correctly. However, too much cholesterol is known to be one of the deadliest factors in the category of health. To give you an example, if you have too much cholesterol, you have more chances for heart attack and stroke. When people talk about overweight or obesity, the main subject is extra fat in the body. So a muscular person could weigh more than an average person. But being muscular and weighing more that way it is alright. We don't want to have too much fat in our body. So if

1: Fit or Fat book by Dr Covert Bailey

people reduce their body fat, then in my opinion, they make themselves healthier[1]. I know that obesity and being overweight, are the mother of a lot of diseases that you don't want to get. For example, cholesterol, excessive production of uric acid, and extra sugar in the blood are caused by being overweight. Now let's talk about uric acid. To some level, your body creates uric acid. There is a normal level for this uric acid. However, if the uric acid level, in your blood, goes above normal, then a disease is caused over some time, which is called gout. When you have gout, you might get a gout attack. Gout attack hits the joints in the body. For example, gout might attack you on the joints, on the toes, etc. this attack is very painful. The pain is so much sometimes say in the knees that you probably will have a very hard time to walk. On the other hand, I know of people who have reduced their uric acid and gout attacks, simply by reducing their weight i.e. reducing the fat contents of their body.

Let me give you an example of a smart eater. This person by proper diet and exercise was able to reduce the uric acid in the body, blood pressure, cholesterol, and drastically reduce the sugar content of their body. For your information, there is a test for checking one of the blood contents, which is called A1C. The A1C test will tell you if you have diabetes, or perhaps, prediabetes. This person that I told you earlier, was able to reduce the A1C to a normal level, and cure himself or postpone diabetes and prediabetes. According to a doctor, as long as you keep your diet and exercise there is no reason for that person to get prediabetes or diabetes. The people who get diabetes by inheritance are a different story. There are many people in this category of a high level of A1C. These people in my opinion could at least reduce the A1C level in the blood or as I said earlier, sometimes they could get themselves to normal blood level i.e. out of prediabetes zone. People with prediabetes, who don't take care of themselves, could easily become regular diabetes. I have not heard of anyone who has diabetes and has been cured of this disease. That is where an intelligent person, will run their annual checkup and see what kind of problems they have. And in the case of people with high A1C or prediabetes, as it is called, I believe they can even cure themselves of this disease or at least reduce the amount of A1C, in their blood, by simply doing the proper diet and exercise.

There is another substance in the blood called HDL. Although HDL, is in the cholesterol family, it is one of the best substances that your body can have. It is called good cholesterol. The more good cholesterol you have in your body the better it is to neutralize the bad cholesterol. It is a known fact that exercise can increase good cholesterol i.e. HDL. As a reminder bad cholesterol is the cause of heart attack, stroke, and who knows how many other illnesses are caused by LDL which is the bad cholesterol. If you are interested in this subject you might ask your doctor to talk about it, in a simple language.

The next not to do in the list is the poison powder that is known in common language as sugar. People love to eat sweet things. But a lot of people don't know that too much sugar is really bad for them. Too much sugar leads to diabetes, and also obesity. However, I believe moderation, is the keyword. If you have no health complications, and you are not overweight, then I guess a little bit of sugar, or sugary foods, here-and-there is alright. As you know there is sugar in soda, all kinds of candy bars, chocolate bars, etc. I must say something about soda that might be interesting to you. I know for example as a general rule all of the sodas have too much sugar is in them. Also, I know of, a lot of people that, every time they drink soda or carbonated beverages get heartburn. There are better alternatives for snacks in my opinion. For example, a few Roasted, unsalted nuts[1], say a handful, along with one count of fruit, could be just as satisfying as a candy bar and soda. Feel free to drink water, even a glass of milk. The fact is that the sugar in fruits due to the fiber contents of the fruits, is less harmful than the table sugar that we all know. The sugar in fruits can be digested and consumed better, and easier. You might take this kind of snack two times a day when you felt hungry or when you have the urge for it. Again it is wise to consider the first principle in "how to tell your body, not to store fat". Apply this when you are taking this snack. So try to eat snacks on time too.

From what I have seen, nowadays a lot of people including young children eat too much sugar. Subsequently, we see a lot of people, even kids with diabetes, or obesity. Another very dangerous complication of sugar is clogged up arteries, according to a vascular specialist doctor. As you might know vascular means of arteries, veins, etc., that carry blood all over the body. The doctor continued, sugar is known to create triglycerides in the blood. Triglycerides are one of the main causes of clogged arteries in some people. The best course of action is to take your annual checkup on time. That way the doctor can advise you as to what to concentrate on. For example, he might ask you to reduce the sugar level because you're getting close to the diabetes border or you are overweight and you need to cut down the sugar, etc. Today we see a lot of people over 50 that have to go through heart surgery or put stents in the arteries that are connected to the heart. I deduct that, the most likely candidate for this problem is sugar. It is a known fact that clogged up arteries could lead to a heart attack. Also, diabetes for many people is caused by too much sugar in the diet. I can tell you some horror stories about diabetes that I have heard. It restricts you if you got it. That means there are a lot of kinds of foods that you cannot eat if you got it. Worse than that is the fact that, people with diabetes might lose limbs, even a whole eye, just to save their lives. The bottom line is, I have heard and seen that diabetes causes early death.

ALERT: Based on my deductions for people over 50. And especially if you are overweight, and have consumed a lot of sugar in the past, I urge you to take a blood test and check your blood sugar level. If this level is high, I deduct that you might have clogged arteries somewhere. Insist on your check-up, and referral to a cardio, or vascular specialist for clogged up arteries. This could save you from heart surgeries, or heart attack. Perhaps your doctor could tell you, that if you have these conditions you might want to check for any specialist that he recommends for you to go to.

HOW IMPORTANT IS WATER?

Water is on the to-do list. According to the Books have read, about 70% of humans' body is water. So I believe water is very important for us. From what I have read also to keep a healthy body, an average adult, must at least drink an average of eight glasses of 10 oz water, per day. A medical doctor also told me, that for people who have constipation, one of the best remedies is water. I know of a lot of people who have tried this and got great results.

1: Fit or Fat a book by Dr Covert Bailey

What I'm trying to emphasize is that, do not discontinue or start taking any medication on your own. For your information, I must emphasize one more time, that I have seen people who discontinued their medication, and had experienced health problems. Once again I confirm do not play around with the dosage, stopping, or starting any kind of medications. Also do not play doctor with your health on your own.

From what I have read in the books, water is very necessary to wash away the chemicals that are created in the body. From what I know, kidneys will function better if you have more water in your body. A lot of you, know this fact, but I have to say it here. I think overdoing anything could be dangerous. Although Water is very necessary for the body, too much water I presume, is not good either. On the other hand, I have read several articles, that indicated that lack of water in the body, could create dehydration. Dehydration is one of the main causes of kidney damage and kidney failure according to the articles that I have read. So this emphasizes, that moderation is the best way to go.

ANOTHER ONE IN THE TO-DO LIST, "DOCTORS"

In my opinion, one of the most important parts of keeping healthy, and losing weight is a very responsible and good doctor. By responsible I mean, the Doctor Who will follow up with you and guides you and Helps to improve your health. In my book, the doctor has the ultimate say in whatever you do, for your health. If you have read, a few good documents, books, or watched, informative videos, etc., does not and must not mean that you take the matters in your own hand without the help of a professional. My reasoning is that the doctors have been educated especially to keep your health. No matter how many books, or articles that, you have read, you might miss a simple but crucial point. The issue is specially when you take any drastic action or start or end any medications. The fact is that; people generally have not been educated for medical science. Even if you miss a little point that you might ignore, it could make the difference between life and death or healthy or unhealthy.

As mentioned before, your doctor has the final say. But you can influence his decision. By influencing their decision, you might be able to persuade your physician to change your prescription or reduce or increase the dosages of the medications that you might or you might not be taking. In some cases, you might influence your physician to disconnect or perhaps even not prescribe some medications for you. Let me start with an example. For the case of this person that I know very much about, he was supposed to take, medications for cholesterol, and blood pressure. Furthermore, this person had a high level of A1C, which is called prediabetes. His doctor told him that all of the symptoms or problems that he has are due to his overweight/or obesity. He made a deal with him, that if he seriously sticks with that diet, the physician had specified, he might consider, to change his prescriptions. That doctor told me, that he has seen a lot of these cases, and he knew if he gives the patient incentive, the patient might even take some of the blood abnormalities of his body, to the normal level. For people with high sugar levels in the blood, there are special exercises that the doctor prescribes. I am not interested to indicate these exercises at this point. That patient, finally lost a lot of weight and reduced his cholesterol, blood pressure, and reduced the A1C in his blood to a satisfactory level. The doctor told me that due to his actions, the patient will not get the medication for cholesterol, or diabetes or any medications for blood pressure. Of course, the doctor will keep a tap, as a responsible doctor, of the whole situation. If the patient's situation changes, he will prescribe different medication, exercises or whatever that is necessary. That's what I mean by influencing your doctor. My suggestion to anybody who reads this section or this book is to always take your annual checkup, and make an appointment with your caring doctor right after the blood test results are sent to you. At that visit, the doctor has to tell you what the deficiencies are, or what you have extra in your blood that might be harmful. At that point, the doctor might prescribe extra vitamins or special medication or whatever that is necessary. A lot of the health practitioners, just suffice with an annual checkup and sending the results to the patient. A lot of these doctors or health practitioners, don't make the patient take an appointment after the blood test or the annual checkup. At this visit, which I call it very important follow up, and is ignored by a lot of people, a lot of things can change. Like I said before, at this meeting the doctor can tell you what you're missing, or what prescription you have to take less or more. I believe that I came up with this idea of a meeting after the blood test, and more often than an annual checkup. Furthermore, for people who are making a change in their lives, I suggest that at the critical moments, that is when the doctor is about to give you cholesterol medicine or blood pressure medicine, etc. try to perhaps for lack of better word religiously follow the diet and exercise and then depending on how much time the doctor will give you, try to take another blood test. Let this affect, and influence your doctor to either give you more time or perhaps change his mind about the medications he was about to prescribe for you. For the case study of that patient that I mentioned a couple of pages ago. The doctor gave him six months to see if he can reduce his weight. At this point I recommended to the patient, to take a blood test, to see better what the results were. Fortunately for the patient, he had improved. So the doctor gave him an additional six months. After the blood test, it was proven to my friend I.e. the patient, that, first of all, he can influence the decision of his doctor, but also not take any blood pressure medication or cholesterol medication. The doctor wants the patient under observation, to make sure that the blood pressure, the cholesterol, and A1C or the blood sugar etc. does not jump all of a sudden. Once again I emphasized to my friend that do not take the matters in your hand. And that he must constantly be in touch with his doctor, to make sure his normal levels of cholesterol, blood pressure, and sugar etc. remain in the healthy range. The happy ending for this patient was that he did not have to take any medications for these illnesses. According to my studies and interviews with doctors, the doctor might change the medications for you or reduce the dosage or maybe even cut down a certain medication totally. All of this accomplished by proper diet and exercise. At this point I must repeat, again and again, keep taking the medications that the doctor gives you, also keep the proper diet and exercise, since your health depends on it. This way you might be able to replace your medications with a healthy diet and exercise or at least reduce the dosage of the medication.

Of course the doctor is the only one to reduce dosage, and cut out a medication from the list of your mediations.

CAUTION : Except regular walking, for any exercises wait 2-2.5 hours after each meal before starting the exercise.

CHAPTER FOUR

Diet

Note: you might want to refer to annex eight titled how to make diet food delicious, after reading this chapter.

DIET, USING SCIENCE.

From what I have learned, the best for your body is three meals per day. Each meal, for an average adult, should contain about 20 to 22 grams of protein in it. Protein can be found in chicken, turkey, beef, fish, etc. Also beans family, like chickpeas, lentils, favabeans, legumes and so on. This family is called a starchy vegetable family. The advantage of starchy vegetables is that they have high fiber content. That reminds me of a conference that I attended, that repeatedly discussed the benefit of fiber. One of the most interesting benefits of fiber is that fiber could neutralize the blood sugar. I won't get into how much fiber you have to eat to neutralize the said amount of sugar in the blood. Suffices to say this is a very interesting advantage of fiber, but go to your doctor or nutritionist. Another benefit of fiber is for digestion systems. Fiber is known to have a great effect on digestion problems, such as constipation and others which I won't discuss here. Let's not confuse starchy foods with starchy vegetables. Starchy foods such as bread or potato, perhaps don't have as much fiber in them, but they have more simple carbohydrates. So starchy foods make you gain weight, but starchy vegetables besides the advantage of high fiber, they don't make you gain weight, as much. Starchy foods such as wheat or rice or potato somewhat curb your appetite, however especially for people without much physical activity, it could cause a person to gain weight. To make the discussion more interesting. Some people like to add butter or some kind of oil to potatoes, or bread. Some people make all kinds of foods like cakes, sweetbreads, etc. and add cream or butter to it too. This matter makes this kind of food i.e. starchy foods in the very high weight gain category. So if I leave the jargon out of the discussion, high fiber is good for you, but less fatty, or sweet, or starchy foods may be better.

For the starchy category of vegetables, like beans, 1 1/2 cups of cooked beans per meal should be giving you about 22 g of protein. As for the meat category, a quarter of a pound of meat, chicken, fish, turkey, etc. should be enough per meal. Let me repeat the principle of a roller coaster that I discussed in the previous chapters, as well as all of the principles found in the "tell your body not to store fat and consume it too." By these rules, my argument is that each meal should have the suggested amount of 22 grams of protein in it. If you go above that or if you go below that or if you starve or indulge, you will put yourself on that roller coaster and fat saving mode. Let me remind you again that, in my opinion, fat[1] must stay out of your diet. By now you should know that your worst enemy is fat. It is not acceptable in the diet, since the fat that you eat can easily turn into body fat[1]. And that body fat is the root cause of a lot of diseases that you don't want. So let me repeat that by fat I mean[1], butter, cooking oil, fried food, chips, and anything that has fat or cholesterol in it. Let me illustrate[1] a fact that it doesn't matter whether it is regular fat or saturated fat or polysaturated fat, they are all bad. So keep fat out of your diet. Also, you should read the label of anything you buy whether munchies or any kind of food, to see if it has fat in it, and if it does, how much fat? Another item that you want to look for on the package of your grocery items, is salt. Salt is sometimes labeled as sodium. Now I want to bring a subject of RDA. As you know RDA means Recommended Daily Allowance. RDA is determined by the United States food and drug administration. It is a list of all of the elements or substances, such as vitamins, proteins, carbohydrates, sodium, fat, etc. that you can take as a maximum per day. So when you look at the package, you read the percentage of RDA value. For a small bag of munchies, for example, if it has more than 5% as a ballpark, of the daily recommended allowance of sodium, or fat then I would say that the item is probably not recommended in my opinion.

So for an average person, a breakfast like milk and cereal or eggs, etc. is alright. Two protein categories of foods, one for lunch and one for dinner should be enough. Now I brought a subject up before, a way that you can eat all you desire and not gain weight. Maybe there is a way. I believe that the green vegetable category of foods will not cause you to gain any weight. Again moderation for fiber foods is recommended. According to a research done too much fiber especially without protein needed, could be harmful. The high fiber foods such as vegetables make your digestive system work harder, and close to all of it will come out, after digestion. A lot of it also, is water and the excess water comes out of your system easily by urinating. So combine the exact amount of protein that your body needs, like mentioned before for average person 22 grams of protein, with a lot of different vegetables. Just to make vegetables tasty you can cook some of these vegetables. For example, broccoli, cauliflower, asparagus, carrots, etc., Can be boiled, or steamed. You can always use all kinds of sauces that are available to add to vegetables to make them tasty. Let me remind you that, before you buy any sauce, you should read the labels. The label will tell you how much fat, salt, sugar, and other substances there are in that jar of sauce. This way you can avoid sauces that contain too much salt, sugar or fat. This way you can enjoy a good meal and have enough nutrition and at the same time keep your proper diet, by adding a lot of vegetables if you desire, to curb your hunger. Note: you might want to refer to annex eight titled how to make diet food delicious, after reading this chapter. I forgot to mention, for vegetables that are awkward to cook such as lettuce, cucumber or green peppers, you can add the vinegar or hot sauce, or combine vinegar and hot sauce and then add it on top of the raw lettuce tomato, etc. This way again you get very tasty vegetables, along with your food.

In the previous chapters, I emphasized, eating fatty foods is not a good idea. Substances such as butter or cooking oil, etc. are not good ideas for a diet, for people who want to lose weight.

1: Fit or Fat a book by Dr Covert Bailey

Fat of any kind in any meal is not a good idea. The best options are boiled, steamed, or oven cooked type of meals. There are so many substances and add-ons in the market that you can buy and combine with steamed vegetables or steamed food or cooked meals and make it tasty for yourself and that's the key point. There are so many sauces that you can make on your own. For example, take some yogurt[1] and add some honey and some hot sauce perhaps. There you go, you have a very tasty sauce for your food. Ketchup, tomato sauce, or all kinds of sauces could be good as long as you keep a moderate amount. I also recommend that you stay away from sauces that have too much fat, salt or sugar. I believe the taste of salt, sugar, and fat can be replaced with different kinds of spices that are available.

Vitamins.

We need vitamins, minerals and all kinds of other substances for our body. I believe, off counter vitamin pills are available. But as long as you read and keep the dosage right, you should be alright. Lack of vitamins and minerals could cause problems. I spoke with a few people, who told me since they had started those multivitamins, they noticed that they were losing weight. According to my experience, taking these vitamin pills say about half an hour before exercise could be very useful in terms of being more energetic and perhaps losing weight.

I also recommend that for snacks, a handful of nuts[1] maybe, plus some milk or cheese and fruit could be a very good snack. If you have a desire for sugar, why not eating a banana or a sweet fruit. Perhaps you can add some raisin to the handful of nuts or add some honey to the nuts and what a delicious snack it makes. I want to remind you that the sugar that you can find in the fruits or honey, due to fiber contents, is better than the sugar powder that you buy from Super Market. The sugar in fruits and honey is better and faster consumed, due to the fiber contents, and According to my investigation and deduction, sugar in the fruits, honey, or raisins, etc., does not create too much triglycerides. I have discussed before that specially with prediabetes, triglycerides are very bad for you, and could cause clogged arteries. A Dr. told me that, sugar is one of the worst substances that creates triglycerides in the blood

Cake and Cookie Lovers

I have a pointer for cake and cookie lovers. Sometimes when I am in the mood for cookies cakes etc. I get a tall glass of 16 oz milk plus some cookies or a medium muffin and then turn this to a meal. It's nutritious and very satisfying. I make sure, the cake categories, do not have too much cream, fat or sugar on it. So, for instance, this could be your lunch, dinner, or breakfast.

1: Fit or Fat a book by Dr Covert Bailey

CHAPTER FIVE

Exercise

CAUTION: For children that are under age, especially under 15 years old, parents' guidance is strongly recommended for this section, for the understanding of heart rate monitor, and all kinds of exercises.

CAUTION: Except regular walking before starting any exercises, wait for 2-2.5 hours after each meal.

Exercise should be a joy for you every time. Exercise could be your best friend that, improves your health and also makes you lose weight. But the proper way of exercise is very important. I always try to keep a good posture during exercise. That means no arches in the back. Also for example for weight lifting, your hands, arms, and forearms must be aligned and parallel to the body while you're doing the exercise. Even the wrist and ankles must be in a straight line and not bent. This way you could avoid getting all kinds of joint pains or back pains in the future. Please refer to annex 5. It gives you some guidance as to how to determine the maximum weight that you can lift or other things that you might need. You might find this annex very useful.

This book is about improving your health and losing weight. I had no intention of this book to be for bodybuilding or people who like to exercise with heavy weights etc. I have seen a lot of people who exercise regularly, and they are much older than they look. However, it must be said that like anything good in the world, if you don't use it properly it could sometimes hurt you. I have heard of stories of old people especially, and even younger people who get a heart attack, and sometimes they get into life-threatening situations during exercise. So once again I like to emphasize that proper exercise is the key. In this chapter, I have tried to show you some ways of proper exercise. I have also indicated some procedures that if you follow I am pretty sure you will be alright. The fact of the matter is that people sometimes either get carried away or they don't feel what they are doing. For example, people respond very well with pain or running out of breath. But things are not that simple, you have to take care of yourself. These procedures that I have found, could make exercise very much harmless and very joyful. Remember if you are suffering during the exercise or you are straining yourself you are doing something wrong. If you're not enjoying your exercise you're doing something wrong. I'm pretty sure I have found myself the safest way to exercise. This way you get a joy and improve your health. I know of people who, exercise regularly and look much younger than they are. The proper exercise gives you, "exercise addiction", best addiction in the world that I know of.

A proper way to exercise

Any exercise that I do, I am always using all of the muscle groups that I can think of, that can be used during exercise.

CAUTIONS: Using all of muscles at the same time may raise your heart rate. Watch your monitor all the time for heart rate, using a small electronic device called Heart Rate Monitor. This monitor can be obtained for about $100.

Obviously, during the whole exercise, you must keep a straight posture. That means no arches in the lower back, middle back, or upper back. Please see figure 1.

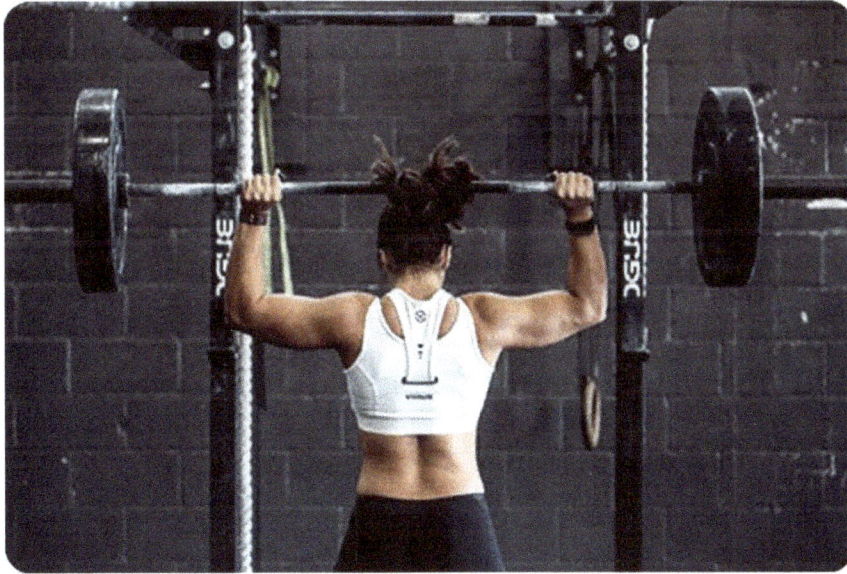

Figure 1 shows this woman during exercise. See how she keeps
her back straight, with no arches in the back.

To do this, that means you are using the calf muscles, both front and back leg muscles, also use your stomach, your buttocks, shoulders, and all of your back. By all of your back I mean the lower back, the mid-lower back, the middle back, the upper middle back, and finally the upper back. Also always keep your wrists and your ankle straight. Let me clarify a little bit, that means whenever you are exercising, try to pressure all of these muscles that I mentioned above, throughout the exercise. To make better use of stomach, it's better to tuck your stomach.

Please see figure 2.

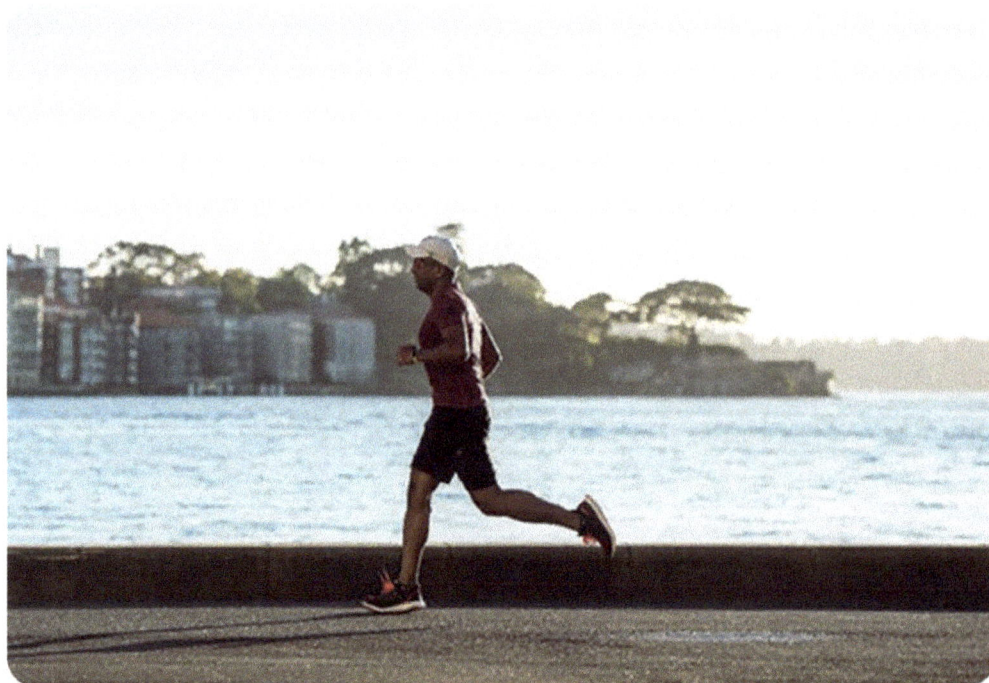

Figure 2 shows this man using all of the muscle groups in his body.

Th is way of exercise needs a lot of practice. For me it took, perhaps a couple of months to adjust myself to this way of exercise. Th e main issue is to practice and keep practicing until you learn. People who are so much out of shape, or maybe due to age considerations, caution is very crucial. Using the heart rate monitor during exercise is very necessary in my opinion. Remember to check the display of the heart rate monitor at least every fi ve seconds. A better way, of course, is to stare at the display of the monitor during the whole exercise.

When you are doing Hard or rigorous exercises, I have a pointer for you. First halt the exercise. You breathe in, and then you force the air out through the mouth. You want to force the air out of the entire lungs as fast as possible. You can repeat a couple of times. Th is will cause all of the carbon oxides, and all the bad stuff to get out of your lungs. This practice of getting all of the air out of your lungs with force is very good even in situations that say you are in a place that there are lots of bad chemicals gases etc. and you have inhaled the bad air. In this kind of situation, go to fresh air maybe outside, then breathe in and force the air out just like specified in the previous lines. This way you get a lot of bad stuff out of your lungs. Obviously, by doing so, a lot of people are known to have their pulse rate dropping a little bit. This is good since as you know when you are doing rigorous or hard exercises your pulse rate is at a high-level.

PLACE OF EXERCISE

A lot of people go to the gym, or they might choose to walk or jog outside. All of these places are well ventilated. However, I have made myself an in-home gym. I have chosen a stationary bike, and some weights to lift. I have turned my dining room into a gym. I ventilate by opening all the windows that I could open. Additionally, I have some fans preferably one for letting air in, and the other to let the air out. The location of the fans should be on opposite sides of the room, i.e. one lets the air in and the other one lets the air out. And there is a distance between these two fans. In cold days I also use central heat or electrical heat. This is necessary since if you have some other ways of heating then I presume they are the kind that consumes oxygen in your room. This consuming the air by the heater is not something that I want. Also, I haven't figured out why, but for some reason whenever I exercise outside in fresh air, my pulse rate goes higher than when I'm exercising at home. So, once again at all times, monitor your heartbeat rate. Please see the following pages that describe the optimum heart rate and how to monitor your heart rate. In my opinion, these following pages are the most important part of this book.

Principle of Optimum Heart Rate[1]

In the books I have read there is a subject called optimum heart rate[1]. Let me tell you the properties of this rate. It is a rate at which you start losing weight[1]. According to the books that I have read, and a doctor confirming this fact, If you don't get your heart rate to this level no matter how much you exercise you will perhaps not get anywhere in terms of losing weight[1], especially losing fat. This means if you can exercise at this heart rate your body will decide to consume the fat[1]. This is the rate that gives you joy. This is the rate that if you go below it, you will not get anywhere in equal time vs someone who observes this rule. At the same time if you go above it you have the possibility of really hurting yourself. A lot of people who cause life threats to themselves, or get heart attacks at the gyms, during exercise, because perhaps they don't know this principle of optimal heart rate. At any age, if you exercise above the optimum rate for too long, i.e. for more than a few seconds, you could cause hurt and life-threatening situations to yourself. I have heard of this fact many times. Optimum heart rate is a fraction of the maximum of the heartbeats that your heart can deliver. For example, the maximum heartbeats of a person could be 150 beats per minute. Then for this case study let's call it, the optimal heart rate could be 125 or something like that. Now I know that somebody can get confused as to how do I know what my maximum is in the first place. Then if I even know that fact, how do I know what the fraction of that maximum is. What is my optimum heart rate finally? The answer is simple. I think it's worthwhile for you to invest in yourself, and pay a cardio specialist to determine your maximum heart rate and finally your optimal heart rate. That's the safest way that I know to determine your optimum heart rate. Especially if you have any heart condition or pulmonary i.e. lung problems or even any kind of health problems, I recommend that you must discuss this with the cardio specialist to determine your optimum heart rate.

21

1: see the book by Dr Covert bailey called Fit or Fat

If you were doing this by yourself all you need is a calculator, also patience to double-check your answers to make sure you have arrived at the right answer. But I still believe you should think that you are worth it, and invest in yourself, and go to a cardio specialist to determine your optimal heart rate by testing. The testing that the doctor does is matched exactly to your body. The formula that I have is sort of like one size shoe fits all, meaning it categorizes the optimum heart rate according to age for an average person. The formula does not consider your health conditions or physical shape. It is based on some average; therefore, you can call it a ballpark estimate of what your actual optimal heart rate is.

Optimum heart rate formula: first you calculate your maximum heart rate, by following a formula. Deduct your age from the number 220. This gives you the maximum heart rate according to your age. Then to determine your optimal heart rate, multiply the maximum heart rate that you calculated, by a fraction. I have read a lot of books, and manuals with different fraction numbers. However, the best way is to categorize people according to their health, and how much out of a shape they are in. For people who are really out of shape, I read, 0.65 is a good start.

For example for a <u>50 year old man or woman</u>
220 − 50 = 170   as you see I subtracted the age from number 220
for an average 50 year old person <u>the maximum</u> heart rate is 170 heart beats per minute.
170 X .65 = 110   here I have assumed this person is out of shape so multiply by .65
For a totally out of shape person in average the optimum heart rate is 110 heart beats per minute.

As your condition improves then you move up to the next level, i.e. the next bigger fraction. The next bigger, the fraction is 0.7, and the one right after that is .75 and as you know .75 is for people who are in relatively good shape. Higher than .75 fraction, I recommend that you consult with a doctor. And finally, the safe, fraction number for the athletes is 0.8. For a very good athlete it could be .85. Sometimes it's hard to monitor and perform at exact optimal heart rate. Therefore, I've come up with a solution. My solution is that I have come up with a range for optimum heart rate this range is two or three heartbeats per minute below and two heartbeats above the optimal heart rate that you got from the formula, or a cardio specialist doctor. For example, for the case study that I discussed for a 50 year old out os shape person , where the optimum heartbeat was 110 Beats per minute, I say as long as you keep your heartbeat between 107 and 112 then you should be alright. As for myself, the moment that my heartbeat goes one beats per minute above the optimum I slow down my exercise. If the heart beat goes 2 beats or more per minute above the optimum, I immediately stop the exercise. Depending on the conditions, you might even decide to sit down for the heartbeat to go down so that you can start over again. That's the best way that I know of, to keep yourself healthy, enjoy your exercise, and finally lose weight and improve your health.

MONITORING THE HEARTBEAT

The best way to determine the heartbeat rate in my opinion is a small electronic device, called a heart rate monitor. A lot of the gyms have this electronic device mounted on some of their exercise equipment. My only problem is that at gyms when you want to do weight lifting or jogging, I don't know how you can monitor your heart rate. A typical value of this electronic device is somewhere around $100 currently. You can purchase this device, from a lot of electronics stores, or sports stores or the Internet. It is simple to use. The one that I have is pretty accurate and I'm very happy with it. The only thing I do, is I wet my chest with water, right on top of the dip on the chest along a strip going from side to side passing through above the dip in the chest. For women wet just below the breasts. That's where the strap of about half an inch wide is placed. You place the strip on the chest area, discussed above, then there is a watch that most likely you will put on your right hand. The watch will tell you exactly what your heartbeat rate is. Some manufacturers have a feature on the watch for heart rate monitor, the moment you go above a set amount say the optimum heart rate, then the watch starts ringing. In that case you need to set the ringer on the monitor.

Another place that I found to put that watch, is on the handlebar of my stationary bike. I used a firm sponge around the handlebar for better strapping of watch and better adjusting and rotating of the watch to see much better. This way I could easily watch the heartbeats without distractions. Even during weightlifting, I can easily take a look at this watch which is on the handlebar. The best way to look is to keep watching every five seconds. Better yet, keep staring at the display during the whole exercise. This way you constantly observe your progress or the heartbeat while you're exercising without halting the exercise. Like I discussed in the previous paragraph, the moment you see your heartbeat rate is above your optimal heart rate, or perhaps with a little tolerance of up to 2 or more bits per minute above the optimal, that's the time you stop immediately. You sit down if the heartbeat is high. Another situation is when your heart rate keeps going up, then it gets close to optimal, maybe a couple of beats per minute before the optimal, in that case, you want to slow down, and keep watching the display.

You adjust your speed, the settings on exercise equipment, or the weight of the dumbbell, etc. until you get to the point that, exercise goes very close to the optimal heart rate, for a good amount of time, without too many halts, or slowing down too much.

Some years ago that we did not have an electronic heart rate monitor, people used to determine their heart beats per minute by a regular watch and placing the right-hand finger specifically the finger next to index finger on an artery that is located on the side of the right of the neck. The pulsating of that artery is the same as the heartbeat. We used to take the pulse for six seconds and count the number of pulses in those six seconds. Then multiply that number of pulses by 10 to get pulses or heartbeats per minute. According to what I have read that's the best place to monitor your heartbeat. That is much better than touching your wrist to get the pulses, or heartbeats per minute. Of course, the heart itself is probably the best source but I presume that is difficult to obtain your heartbeat by accessing your chest, in the middle of your exercise. But then again I must emphasize since you don't have to halt your exercise to measure your heartbeat, the best way is, to buy the Electronic heart rate monitor. Although using the monitor is a simple task, for some people it might be difficult to figure out how to work the monitor or how to set up your heart rate monitor. In these cases, first, consult with the manual that comes with the heart rate monitor. Usually, you could call the manufacturer of that heart rate monitor for questions that are hard to figure out from the manual or maybe the answer is not in the manual. Whether you use the manual or call the manufacturer, you must know how to work the heartbeat monitor. Some manufacturers have a feature on the watch that if you go beyond a limit that you set, then the watch starts ringing. Be careful when you set this limit on the monitor, to set the optimum heart rate or perhaps 2 beats per minute extra. When you hear this ringer you must stop the exercise.

Another caution, if your heart rate on the display is something funny such as a very low number like 30 bpm then you know there is something wrong. For an average person, the heartbeats should be between 60 to 100 beats per minute, at resting time i.e. when you are sitting down or doing nothing. At the resting time, if you see a very low number or very high number of beats per minute on display, first stop the exercise. It could be that the battery is out, or the strap on your chest is not tightened enough. If the strap is not loose then, there's a chance that your chest is dry. That is the time you apply the water on your chest and tighten the strap and start over. Sometimes the low number or no display indicates a weak battery, must be changed.

My idea for senior citizens and people with a health condition: I have an idea for a special group of people. I am about to reveal a deduction or perhaps a theory for senior citizens and people who might have health conditions such as heart conditions. Of course, the word and advice of a doctor is priority number one, and you must consult with the doctor about this theory and whatever you see here. Heart rate monitor device is best to have even during the non-exercise moments. I have heard stories that people who have gotten heart attack during dancing, or getting excited with friends or walking faster than usual, or maybe even during intimate relations with a spouse. This is especially happening with the elderly, or people with a serious heart condition. Perhaps it could happen to anyone, that I don't know and that's a good question to bring up with the doctor. By obtaining this electronic device and constantly observing the watch, that tells you the heart rate. Then you can have it on for any physical activity. Physical activity like walking, dancing gathering with friends that will end up in some kind of physical activity or even intimate activities with the spouse. I think if you know how to program the watch to ring when your heart rate is above the optimum, is a very good idea. I suggest this category of people, to be on the lookout for alarm ring, or watch the display, etc. Then the moment you see or hear that your heartbeat goes higher than it supposed to go, you could stop and maybe this way some people can save their lives. So people who have a loved one that is a senior citizen and or has some kind of health condition specially the heart, they can provide that person with a heart rate monitor and teach them how to use it.

Sub chapter 5-1

Weight Loss cycle

I have found out that, Weight loss has a special cycle. I would rather explain this cycle that I discovered personally, in the following pictures.

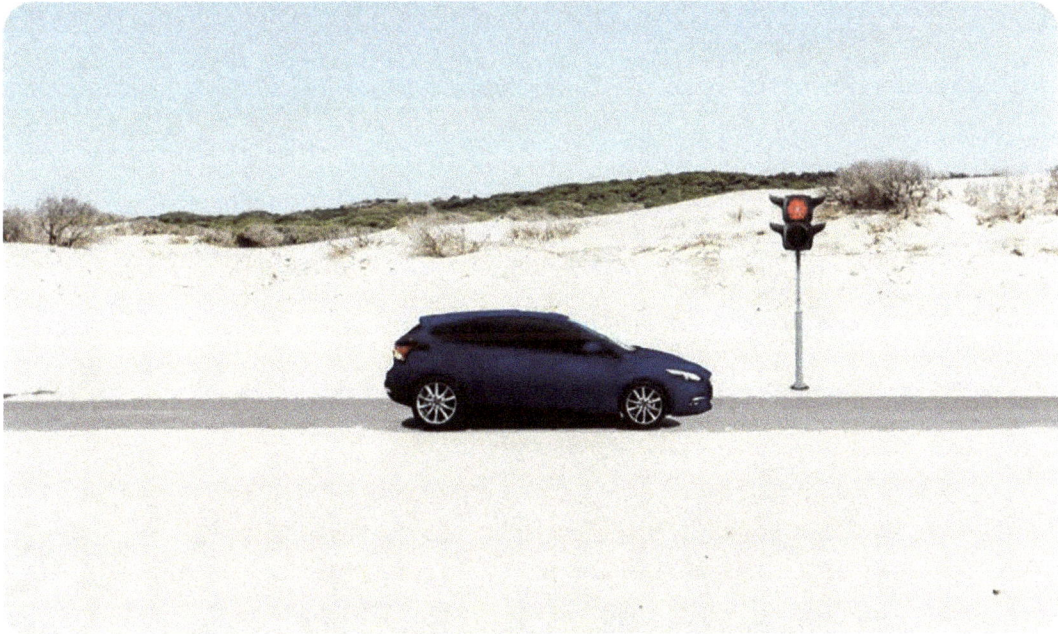

Figure 3: shows by association that for the first few days that when
you start diet and exercise, you will not lose weight. You are stopped.

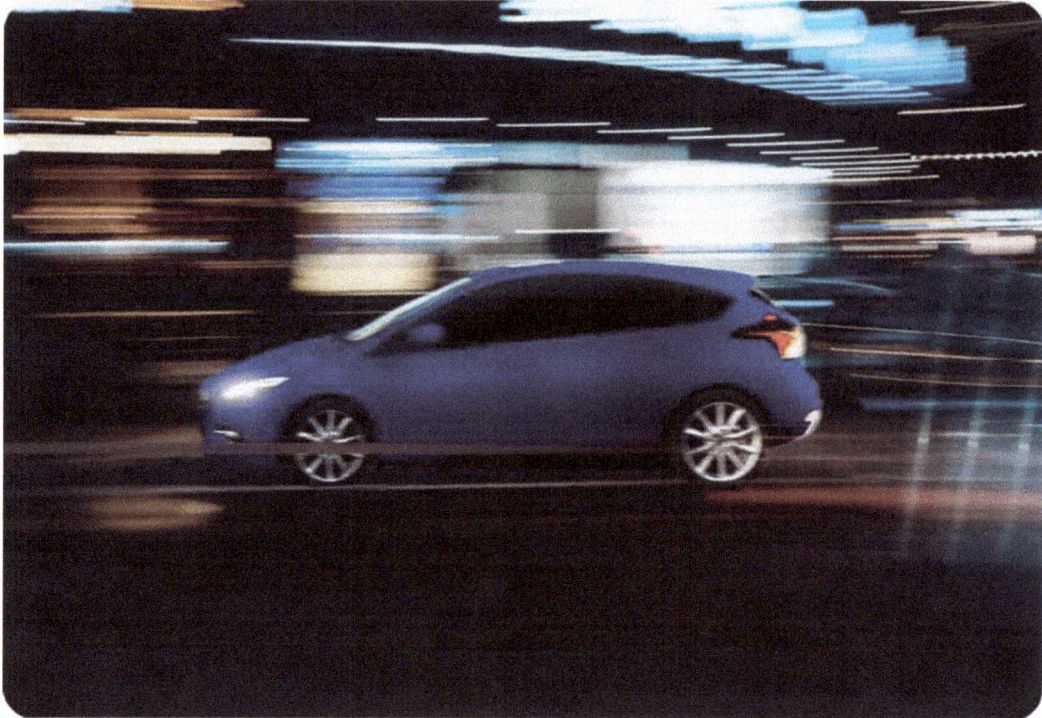

Figure 4: by association shows after a few days of regular exercise and
diet, you would start losing weight, as if you are on fast track.

Let's say that's your first day which I call it the start point. Please look at the pictures. As you can see in figure 3, at the beginning there is a no progress period. This period represents the following days after the starting point. Although you are observing all of the diet and exercise rules, you are not losing any weight. This trend goes on perhaps depending on a person for a few days. This period is in average 2 weeks. Picture 4 is a point called the beginning of weight loss. At this point, you start losing weight. And this trend goes on and on and on and pretty much you lose weight for a while. However, after a few days of weight loss, you probably find yourself in the next graph. Please see picture 5 below, that you are losing weight similar to the fast moving car. Then all of a sudden you stop losing weight. Please see figures 5 and 6.

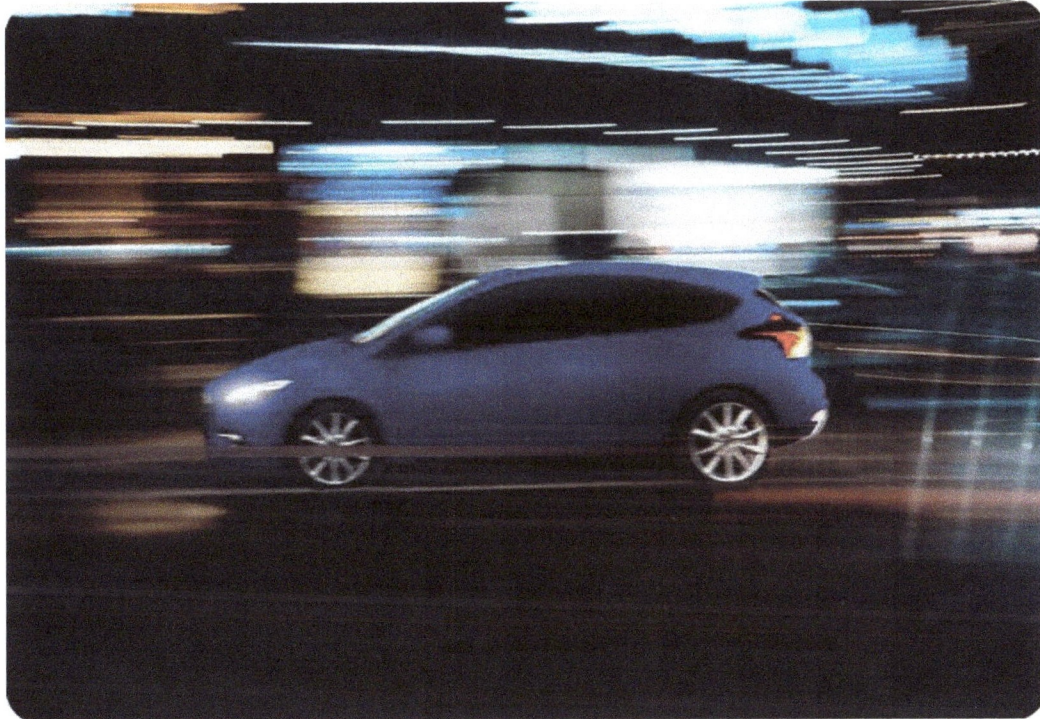

Figure 5: represents that you are enjoying weight loss but see figure 6.

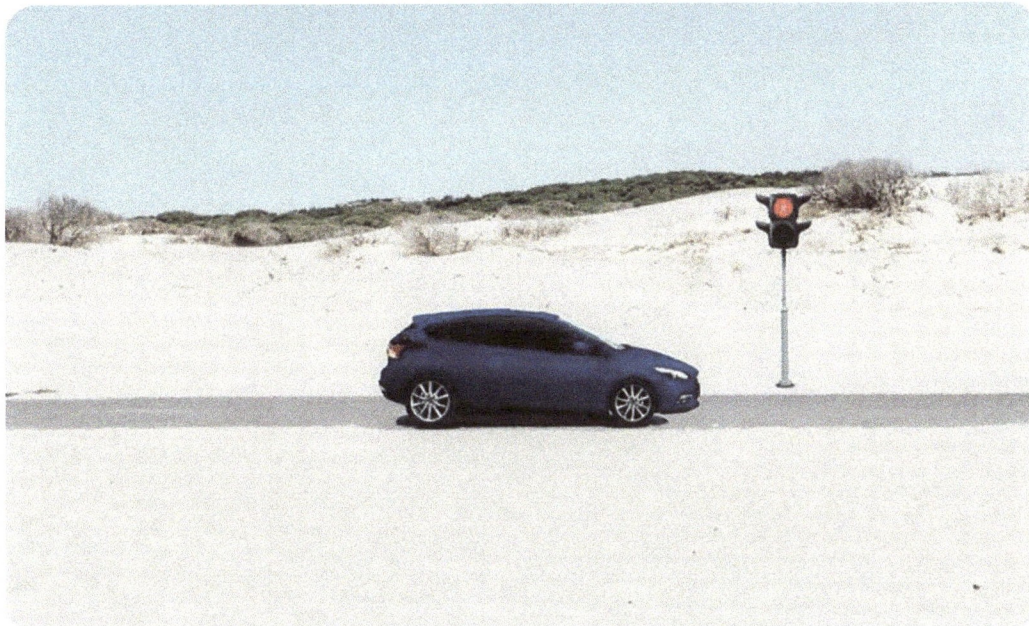

Figure 6 shows that weight loss is stopped, after a few days of weight loss.

As you see you get to the point of weight loss stop, here. This means that you will not lose any more weight at this point for the next following days. This period indicated by the car at stop.

sign. So for the next few days, although you keep your diet and exercise regularly, as you should, you'll find out that your weight is constant and it will not change. But not to worry as you progress you will see yourself again on the weight-loss period. Please see the next Paragraph that shows you how things keep going on and on.

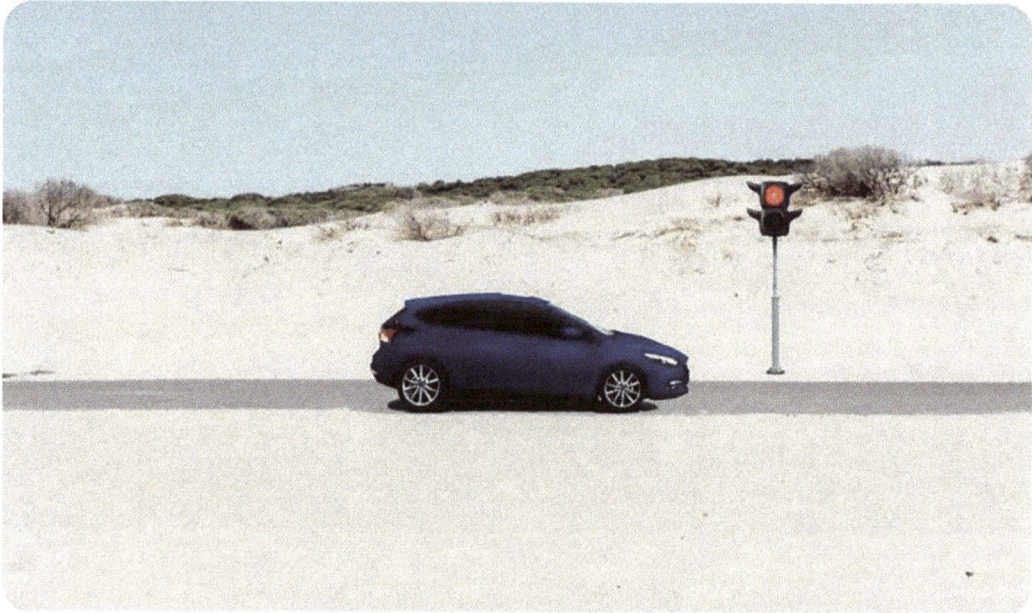

Figure 7: Although you have lost weight in the past few days, you will not lose weight any more. You are stopped.

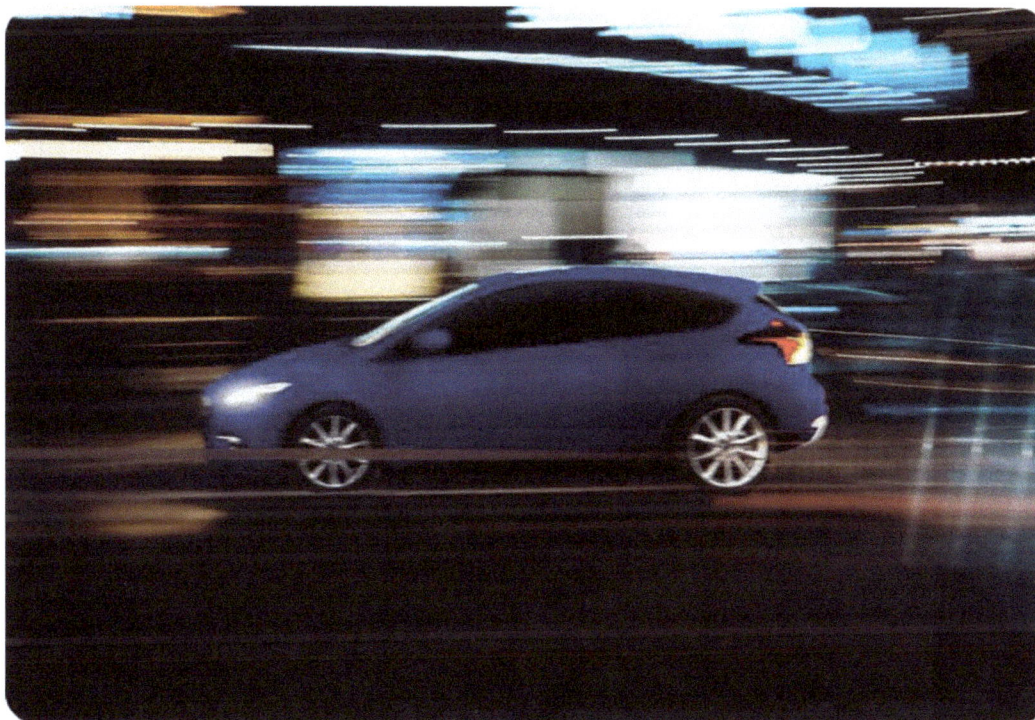

Figure 8: shows after a few days of regular exercise and diet, you
would start losing weight, again on fast track.

As you can see for yourself again, you experience that, the weight loss stops again as shown in figure 7. The stoplight in front of the car shows you that, you are going nowhere with weight loss. That means that for the next few days you will not lose any weight, although you have observed all of the diet and exercise rules. Finally, weight loss starts again. For me, the stop period is usually a week maybe 10 days. The moving on the fast track part indicating weight loss, is usually as much as six or seven pounds. I think a lot of you now get the point.

You will go without any weight loss for some time, although you keep your diet and exercise regularly. And then the weight loss starts then stops again and then starts again. I have personally lost about, a little less than 80 pounds. And throughout this time I saw what happened in terms of my weight and weight loss. I have probably gone through 10 of these Diagrams for 80 pounds of weight loss. The thing is that, you want to act like a train constantly going and going. You don't want to act like an airplane always in a rush to go from one point to the other. Rushing in my belief causes you to run out of breath after a short while and then you get nowhere.

—◁▷—

Subsection 5-2 Exercises

For people over the age of say thirty-five, I urge you to take your blood test before and after the weight loss program. Especially if you are successful to lose a lot of weight, and you were overweight at the beginning you will observe a lot of improvement in terms of your health. Previously I mentioned that, in terms of keeping your social status, sometimes you will have to break your diet. There are also circumstances that you might not be able to exercise on a particular day. For these days, I have suggested something in the earlier pages. See chapter one, under heading: "breaking diet and exercise". Also, I like to emphasize what I have said so many times throughout this book, do not forget to monitor your heart rate no matter what kind of exercise you do.

Walking

Walking is one of the best exercises that I know of. Some people say that I don't want to sweat, or I don't want to exercise so hard. For this kind of people, I have a suggestion you can still lose a lot of weight but it must be a long walk every day. I'm thinking of maybe 1.5 or 2 hours walking every day is not bad. However, if you use the following paragraph as guidance the way I did. You might find that you will lose a lot more weight.

An efficient way of walking

I have come up with a new way of walking, that I have personally tested, I know it could be a very effective way of exercise and losing weight. I am using all of the muscle groups that I can think of, during walking. Obviously, during the whole exercise, you must keep a straight posture. That means no arches in the lower back, middle back, or upper back. A very intelligent way of using your feet and legs, to accomplish faster speed and better exercise.

The first subject is how to gain faster speed by using a smarter way of walking. Please see the picture below, for illustration.

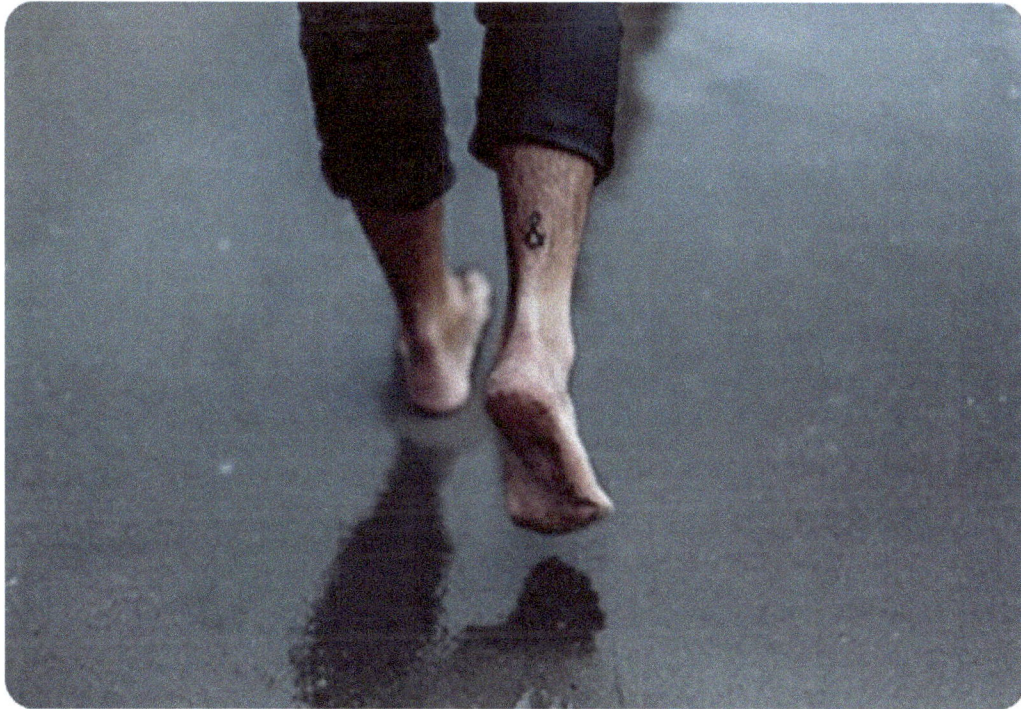

Figure 9: shows how the right foot is about to be thrown forward.

You place one foot forward. Keep the ankles straight. Then let the placed foot to land, on the entirety of the foot. Then you give a push by the entire foot to accomplish the speed, simultaneously with the push, you place the other foot and do the same, as described above. However, it needs a lot of practice at home so that, maybe you take your time, learn at home until you are ready.

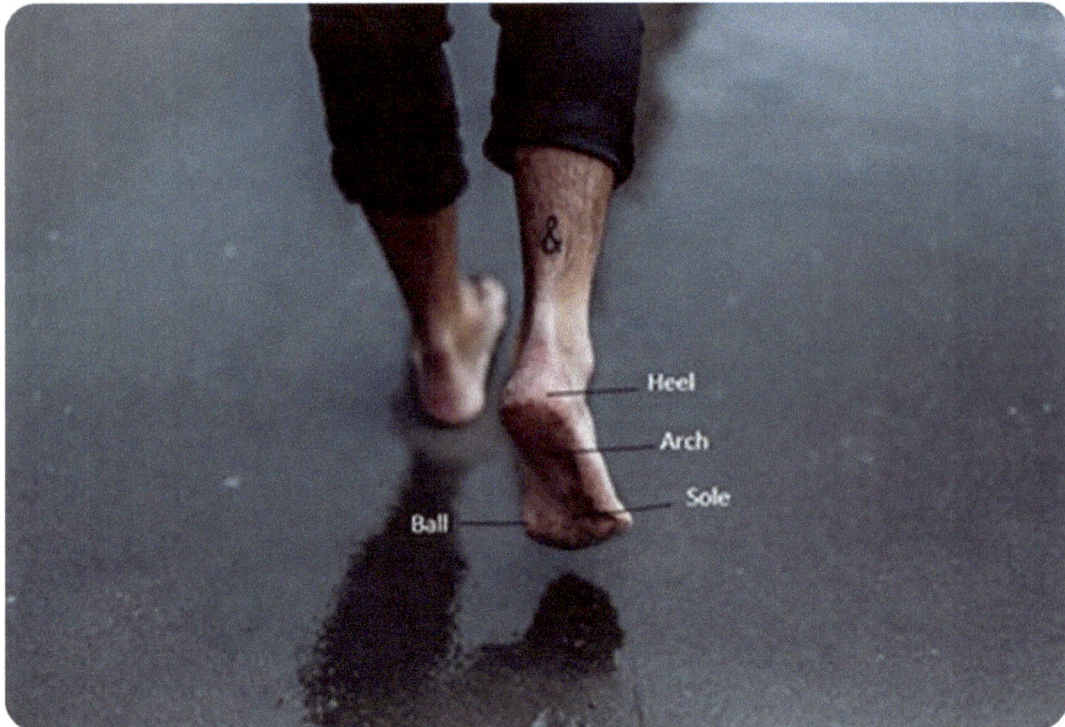

Figure 10 shows different parts of the foot.

The next portion of this new way of walking is a little bit harder for people who don't know about it. It needs a lot of practice.

For me, it took perhaps a couple of months to adjust myself to this way of walking. That's when you use all of the muscle groups that you can use to help you achieve the fast motion, and fat consuming mode. Obviously, during the whole exercise, you must keep a straight posture. That means no arches in the lower back, middle back, or upper back. To do this, that means you are using the calf muscles, both front and back of the leg muscle. Use, your stomach, your buttocks, your shoulder and all of your back. By all of your back I mean the lower back, the mid-lower back, the middle back, the upper middle back, and finally the upper back. Also always keep your wrists and your ankles straight. Let me clarify a little bit, that means whenever you are exercising, try to pressure all of these muscles that I mentioned above, throughout the exercise. To make better use of stomach, it's better to tuck your stomach in. if your hands are free you could swing your hands and arms in harmony with your walking.

CAUTION: This method of walking could raise your heart beat high. Make sure you have the heart rate monitor on, and look at the display every 5 seconds at least. Use caution.

This could be a very rigorous exercise. Although some people, might ask that, how can you believe this simple walking is this much vigorous? The answer is, since you are using more muscles than before, your heart has to work harder to accommodate. By doing this, your body requires a lot more nutrition to these new muscles and oxygen too. If you use all of these muscles at the same time it will raise your heartbeat more than you can think. You might even reach above the optimum heart rate. I have tested these with heart rate monitor several times. Each time I test this I come up with the same conclusion, this gets the heartbeat way up. Of course, for people up to the age of maybe 50, this may not be as bad as senior citizens even 50 years old and younger may find this very rigorous and may find it hard to do. Again I must emphasize it takes a lot of practice at home by yourself to make sure you're doing it right.

---◆◆◆---

Fast walking

Walking is one of the best exercises that I know of. If your speed is good enough, and therefore you get your heartbeat rate to the optimum, that could be considered a very good exercise. Just as I mentioned in the previous pages, you must take caution not to overdo it. I know some people are so much out of shape, or maybe due to age considerations, for them, caution is very crucial. So taking the heart rate monitor with you during fast walking is very necessary in my opinion especially for the groups that I mentioned above.

---◆◆◆---

Cold Stricken Problem

I experienced and discovered the cold stricken problem. I spoke with a doctor, a few years ago. Th e doctor could not diagnose a patient i.e. my old roommate, as to what was causing all of these symptoms with the roommate. The Doctor finally, said there was nothing wrong with the patient. After I took the roommate home, I told the roommate that I call this problem, cold stricken. I came up with this name on my own. The best solution is some heat therapy. i.e. an extra warm blanket during bed time and perhaps a higher level of temperature in the house. Additionally you could buy hot bottle water from the pharmacy or Internet. This hot water bottle can be placed under the blanket when you sleep. I have seen especially senior citizens get cold stricken problem. In this section, I'll bring the symptoms of the cold stricken problem. You might have one or more of the symptoms.

Word of caution: if you have any symptoms of any disease, I recommend you contact your doctor or an emergency room.

The symptoms are as follows. Chest problems such as burning chest, a little bit of runny nose, Shivering, lack of flexibility all over the body, as if your whole body is stiff , a bit of headache and so on. You may have one or more of these symptoms. I want to remind you that if you have any symptoms of any discomfort or illnesses, you must immediately go to a doctor. Let the doctor diagnose you and then if there was no bad diagnosis maybe you can continue with the heat therapy.

The conclusion I made from all of this is that I shouldn't jog the days that the temperature is below tolerance, or especially when there is the wind blowing or there is a very low temperature or wind chill factor, according to the weather forecast. If you are planning to exercise in a cold day the best way is to go to a gym or have a heated home gym.

—◆—

Jogging

Jogging is a very good exercise. As I mentioned before like any other exercise, when you jog, you use all of the muscle groups that you can use to help you achieve the fastest speed, and fastest fat consuming mode.

CAUTION: Thi s method of jogging could raise your heart beat high. Make sure you have the heart rate monitor on, and look at the display every 5 seconds at least.

Obviously, during the whole exercise, you must keep a straight posture. Th at means no arches in the lower back, middle back, or upper back. To do this, that means you are using the calf muscles, both front and back of the leg muscle. Use, your stomach, your buttocks, and all of your back, plus the shoulders. By all of your back I mean the lower back, the mid-lower back, the middle back, the upper middle back, and fi nally the upper back. Also always keep your wrists and your ankle straight. Let me clarify a little bit, that means whenever you are exercising, try to pressure all of these muscles that I mentioned above, throughout the exercise. To make better use of stomach, it's better to tuck your stomach in. You could swing your hands and arms in harmony with your jogging. Th is could be a very rigorous exercise. Although some people, might ask that, how can you believe that, simple jogging that I have done easily in the past, turns to so rigorous, that I must use plenty of caution, watching the heart rate monitor every 5 seconds. Th e answer is, since you are using more muscles than before, your heart has to work harder to accommodate. By doing this, your body requires a lot more nutrition to these new muscles and oxygen too. If you use all of these muscles at the same time it will raise your heartbeat more than you can think. You might even reach above the optimum heart rate. I have tested these with heart rate monitor several times. Each time I test this I come up with the same conclusion that the heartbeat goes way up. Of course, for people up to the age of maybe 50, this will not be as bad as senior citizens. Even people below age of up to 50 years old may find this very rigorous and may find it hard to do. Again I must emphasize it takes a lot of practice by yourself to make sure you're doing it right.

I know in fact by testing and testing it on others too, that if you especially use your buttocks into jogging your speed will go up, i.e. you will run faster.

Please see the cold stricken subheading and a related text for cold stricken. The conclusion I made from all of this is that, best for me is, not to jog the days that the temperature is the below tolerance, or especially when there is the wind blowing or there is a very low wind chill factor according to the weather forecast. If you're planning to exercise, in cold days, the best way is to go to a gym or have a heated home gym.

—◆—

Interesting Complications of Weight loss

I have personally experienced that, extra fat in the body makes you more resistant to cold temperatures. I know of some other people who have experienced the same things. The implication of that is, when you lose weight especially when you lose a lot of weight, you will feel the cold much worse than in your old days that you were overweight.

Also, people who lose a lot of weight could experience joint pains such as the joints on the wrists, which is very temporary. This pain or discomfort will go away soon enough.

I hope that you have found this book interesting so far. Please look at the following annexes that might be interesting to you. Finally, I hope that you see what I have discussed for diet and exercise. Pay more attention to danger, i.e. fat or oily deposits all across. This can kill a lot of people. I think you will enjoy your diet and exercise, and you will see the fireworks as a result.

SECTION TWO

ANNEXES

For very young, to adult men and women of up to maturity age

Caution: For children that are under age, especially under 15 years old, parents' guidance is strongly recommended for the understanding of heart rate monitor, and all kinds of exercises.

Do you want to become taller

For this group of age, I have some exciting news. I bring up a question. Can you make yourself taller? The answer is, under some restrictions yes. It is a known fact that tallness is primarily, determined by genetics. That means if you are not happy about your height, it depends primarily on relatives. Perhaps you have inherited it. That determining genes of a family member might even be your great grandfather's. For example, you might be a short height child in a family of say medium height people, so all of your brothers and sisters might be medium height. Even your parents, in this hypothetical example, have medium heights. Then this hypothetical person might wonder why he or she is short. The answer might be from one of your grandparents, or even great grandparents' short height. The answer to all of these situations is found in the study of genetics and is beyond the context of this book.

I know a lot of you might ask that, do I need to take any hormones or any funny substances such as complicated and very expensive drugs. The answer to this question is no. So yes you can increase your height and no, you don't need to take anything such as hormones or any expensive medications.

According to what I have seen you can still grow taller. For men and women the ceiling age where growth stops is maturity age. The issue of genetics is an important factor in this matter. But the issue of diet and exercise are also important parts. The rich contents of milk plus one of the so called once a day multivitamins are, in my opinion the best way to go.

Milk takes a long time to take effect for you to grow taller but it is very effective. I think However, if you are say teen ager up to maturity age you still have time. the best age probably is before or around age 15 years old. Again it is also important, that you don't overdose or overdo anything definitely not on any drugs even if they are over the counter multivitamins. You must take this matter very seriously. Overdosing multivitamins is dangerous and causes harm.

Observe the dosage of vitamins very seriously. If you are in a hurry to get results fast, you should consult your doctor as I said before. You want the doctor that you feel comfortable with, and you obey everything he, or she says. You also want to do exactly what the doctor says in terms of the dosage and how long you are supposed to take these pills. I have seen a young teenager, who took this diet and multivitamin, on the supervision of a caring doctor, and he was very happy to see that he got to his desired height. I have a suggestion for coffee drinkers. Instead of cream use milk. Use 1/2 of cup of coffee, fill the other half with milk. For children, drink tea. Tea that is not strong is harmless and refreshing. Take 1/2 of cup of tea, fill up the other half with milk. It is very delicious.

There was a researcher that was informed in the subject of growing height. He told me that, doing exercises that cause you to stretch your legs, and the entire body, could also help, with the process of growing taller. Exercises such as volleyball, basketball, etc. regularly, could help you according to this researcher. I have observed that heavy free weight lifters on average are shorter.

As I mentioned before, seems like younger people love to eat sweets and snacks or sweet foods not to mention fatty or salty foods. A lot of younger people are overweight or have obesity problems. I have also heard that a lot of people have prediabetes or diabetes. I like to ask you to read for example chapter 1 which tells you how to tell your body not to store fat and consume the fat too. For example, chapter four shows you the proper diet, it also includes, a delicious snack that you might take two times a day for example. This specified snack used moderately, should not give you prediabetes, or diabetes. A pinch of raisins, for example, could make the snack sweeter. The sugar in raisins is consumed faster and doesn't stay in your body due to high fiber contents of raisins. Don't forget sodas. A lot of beverages that are in the market have too much sugar in them. I urge you to read up on the amount of sugar that there is in one can of soda. There is a lot more I suggest you read all of these chapters and annexes.

Just a precaution, especially children, and senior citizens try to avoid any exercise, except walking in cold days. On cold days, walking may be alright, if the roads are not icy, and the weather is not too cold you must have enough warm clothes even for simple walking. Otherwise, you are liable to catch pneumonia, at any age. Pneumonia can be life-threatening especially for children and seniors.

FOR CHILDREN, PREVENT DIABETES, OBESITY, ETC.

If children or anybody for that matter, eat too many sweets snacks or too much sodas especially if a person is overweight, ask your parents for a blood test. The blood test will tell you if your sugar levels are too high for example or you have too much cholesterol. At this point the doctor will instruct you what to do.

ANNEX TWO

...   tell your body not to store fat and consume it too"

First Principle

First principle is based on the biological clock in our body. In simple terms, the body expects things to happen regularly and on time. That means you should eat every day at the same time for every meal. Also, exercise the same amount every day on time. This way you will help losing weight, and not storing fat. See chapter one.

Second Principle

The second principle is called the roller coaster principle. Do not ride on a weight-loss roller coaster. There are people that, don't eat at all or eat so little in one day and then another day they eat so much. This is like riding a roller coaster. That means you end up gaining more fat, and gain weight. For more details, please see chapter 1.

Third Principle

A person can't always keep their diet. When you go out to eat a lot of food, or foods that are not diet, or if you don't do your regular exercise, then a few hours or at the maximum several hours afterwards you need to increase your exercise for one time. I recommend say one hour of rigorous exercise like jogging or bike riding or a stationary bike the next few hours. There are more details in chapter 1

Fourth Principle

Activate, or reactivate as many muscles, that you usually don't use in exercises, including regular everyday walking. Common improvements, include putting your back and your buttock and every other muscle that you can think of during each exercise. As always make sure you check your heart rate. Since when you put a lot of muscles into an exercise that causes your pulse to go way up. Chapter one has a lot more details.

Fifth Principle

Although especially strong coffee and too much of coffee, could be harmful to your health but based on the fact that, coffee excites the body all over, and hence the muscles, there might be a benefit here. Tea has a lot less caffeine in it. From what I have heard and seen and experienced, tea is not bad for children of a young age, provided that, it's not very strong.

The caffeine in tea or coffee for adults gives you an edge for exercise and work. See annex three for more details.

Principles of "…tell your body not to store sugar in the blood, and consume it too"

First Principle

Fibers are found abundantly in vegetables and fruits. Fibers neutralize the sugar in the blood. See chapter one for details.

Alert: For people with diabetes, or prediabetes fruits are not suitable. Only non-sweet or green vegetables may be suitable. You must consult with your doctor.

Second Principle

Use other kinds of sugars. The best sugar substitutes that I know of are the ones that are found in fruits, Honey and raisins. From what I understand, due to fiber contents of the menioned substances these kinds of sugars are consumed better and faster, and therefore they won't easily stay in the blood. See chapter 1 for details.

Third Principle

When you exercise you consume more sugar, that otherwise, would've been stored in your blood. See chapter 1 for more details.

Principle of optimum heart rate[1]

Optimum heart rate, is the heart rate, in beats per minute, at which you will start to lose weight[1], improve your health, and lets you to hold on to your youth longer. You need a small device called Heart Rate Monitor (HRM). HRMs are around 100 dollars. Please see chapter five. Also see optimum heart rate range in that chapter.

1: Optimum Heart rate: in a book by Dr Covert bailey called Fit or Fat

ANNEX THREE

TEA AND COFFEE

Strong coffee, and too much coffee in a day, could be harmful to your health. But based on the fact that coffee excites the body all over, and hence the muscles, there might be a benefit here. I have found out based on my personal experience, that a little coffee could gives you some kind of agility for walking, working, use of your hands, feet, and legs, etc. I do not recommend coffee for people underage. But tea and Coffee have caffeine in them. The difference is that tea has a lot less caffeine in it. From what I have heard and seen and experienced, tea is not bad for children of a young age, provided that, it's not very strong. Some people even say that tea is also is refreshing, and also it soothes the nerves. So next time you want to exercise perhaps you have just a very little amount of coffee for adults or a small cup of tea for children and see how it works for you. You can check and see if you are more agile and if it is easier for you to exercise or work. What I mean is perhaps it's a good idea to put this coffee or tea whatever is applicable, into the test and see if you get a small edge when you want to work or exercise.

Caution: caffeine in tea or coffee, could raise blood pressure from what a couple of doctors told me.

ANNEX FOUR

Cold Stricken problem

I have discovered this problem. The doctor that diagnoses you, might not find anything wrong with you. I came up with this name on my own. The best solution is some heat therapy. i.e. an extra warm blanket and perhaps higher level of temperature in the house. Additionally, you could buy hot bottle water from the pharmacy or Internet. This hot water bottle can be placed under the blanket when you sleep. I have seen especially senior citizens get cold stricken problem.

―――

Symptoms of cold stricken problem

In this section, I'll bring the symptoms of cold stricken problem. You might have one or more of the symptoms. Word of caution: if you have any symptoms of any disease, I recommend you contact your doctor or an emergency room, as fast as possible. Another precaution, especially children, and senior citizens try to avoid any exercise, except walking in cold days, if road conditions are not icy or slippery, and weather is not too cold. On cold days you must have enough warm clothes even for simple walking. Otherwise, you are liable to catch pneumonia at any age. Pneumonia can be life-threatening especially for children and seniors.

Th e symptoms of cold stricken are as follows. Chest problems such as burning chest, a little bit of runny nose, Shivering, lack of fl exibility all over your body, as if your whole body is stiff , a bit of headache, change of voice, especially stronger voice, and so on.

Caution: if you have any symptoms of any discomfort or diseases, you must immediately go to a doctor. Let the doctor diagnose you and then if there was no diagnosis for any ailment maybe you can continue with the heat therapy.

Th e conclusion I made from all of this is that, I shouldn't do any outdoor exercises, when the temperature is below tolerance, or especially when there is the wind blowing or there is a very low wind chill factor temperature, according to the weather forecast. If you're planning to exercise the best way is to go to a gym or have a heated home gym.

BACK EXERCISES

Making good posture requires, developing muscles in the back. I have come up with a new way of exercising that I have personally tested, I know it could be a very effective way of exercise and losing weight. You are using all of the muscle groups that you can think of, that can be used during exercise. By doing so, you will develop newer stronger muscles in those newly activated muscles. The more muscle you have, the more fat you consume, and less fat that you store in the body. There are lots of concerns with any activity that involves the back. People who don't know the rules could end up with a lot of back ailments that they don't know. One of the worst problems is the abnormalities of the discs on the back. I believe the medical term is the disc hernia. Obviously, during any exercise, you must keep a straight posture. That means no arches in the back i.e. lower back, middle back, or upper back. Try to put all of your back into exercise, your buttocks, front and back leg muscles, calf muscle, stomach, and shoulders too. To do this try to put pressure on the muscles mentioned. You should feel that you are pressuring the muscles. Your back has 5 parts in my opinion, but I usually have read 3 parts, i.e. lower back, middle back, and upper back in the books. I have found out that the middle back actually has 3 parts i.e. lower middle, middle and upper-middle back.

Caution: your heart rate goes up, by using more muscles, I would observe the heart rate monitor at least every 5 seconds during exercises. See chapter 5 for the heart rate monitor. Th is is seriously important. Th e reason is, since you are using more muscles than before, your heart has to work harder to accommodate. By doing this, your body requires a lot more nutrition to these new muscles and oxygen too. If you use all of these muscles at the same time it will raise your heartbeat more than you can think. You might even reach above the optimum heart rate. Remember it is never too late to strengthen the back muscles. But if you start at a young age you will be doing yourself a great favor. This way you won't have arches in the back when you're standing, sitting or walking.

Back twist problem

Be very careful, when you are doing back exercises including picking up some weight from the floor, you always align your back and your entire body on a straight line i.e. your back should not be at any angle with respect to your lower body. Your upper part and your lower part should be aligned in a straight line. Do not lift weight or box from left to right or vice versa. Walk to the box, make sure your upper and lower body are aligned, then walk to left or right. When you have a weight on your hand, don't twist or turn your back to do the job, even if the weight is as light as 5 lbs. When you have a box or a weight in your hand you don't turn your upper body out of alignment with respect to your lower body. As I said before it is best to walk to the left or right and don't let your back do the job. Please see the following figures to show you the right way to pick up something from the floor or even moving some object while your back is straight.

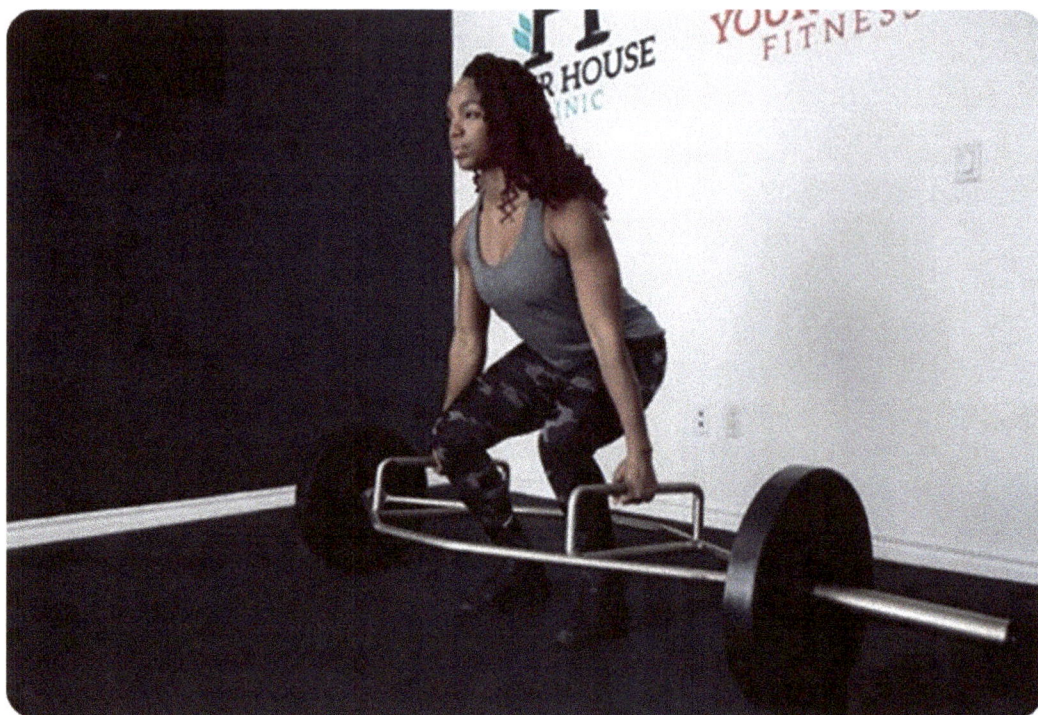

Figure 11 shows this woman puts ½ of the load of the back on the knees
by bending the knees. Also she keeps the back straight.

The second thing you want to remember is that when you want to pick up something from the floor you must bend your knees. This way you will put half of the load on your back and the other half on your knees. You must remember that the back is very sensitive and must be handled with extreme caution. People who don't take enough caution when they are lifting something they might end up with disc hernia which is very likely to be permanent damage to the back. Some people with disc hernia might have to go to surgery to even be able to relieve their pain. The bad part about it, is that when you are doing it you don't feel that, you are doing something wrong until one day after repeated mistakes of lifting the wrong way, some people get real back pain. From then on it might be bad news. Some careless or unaware people, get back pain for the rest of their lives. Please see the figure above for the proper way of lifting something from the floor that shows you the person has bent her knees and keeping her back straight i.e. free of any kind of arches. Also during lifting or moving anything around, do not turn your waist i.e. upper and lower back must be in a straight line

The back twist exercise, is done with a very lightweight object. I use a dumbbell weighing

2.5 pounds. For underage, I recommend that you do not do this exercise. You want to consult with your gym teacher or your chiropractor or your orthopedist doctor to give you the maximum weight that you can use for this exercise. While you're holding the 2 ½ pounds weight with both hands, your arms are extended, below your stomach. Then you try to twist from one side to the other, going as far as you can go using your waist. You can repeat this say 10 times to the left, 10 times to the right.

A N N E X   S I X

FOR PEOPLE 50 AND UP

I was told by a doctor, that at age 50, men or women start getting all kinds of Health problems. I was told also that the best thing to do, is to listen to your doctor. Take doctor's advice as priority number one compare to the advice you get from other sources of information, as a general rule.

At the beginning of the book I mentioned that this rule is very true, however by doing proper exercise and diet, you might be able to influence your doctor into a better decision. For example, by diet and exercise, as I was told by another doctor, you improve your blood pressure or cholesterol or other things, you might be able to influence the doctor's decision to give you a different dosage or in some cases maybe even take out a drug out of your life. I have observed this matter personally. Here is a suggestion, take your check-up as usual as ordered by your doctor, and then start on this diet and exercise that is recommended by this book. Then after a few months, maybe six months or a year take the blood test and ask your doctor if you have made any improvements. I have seen a lot of people who are shocked by doing this, and observing how much their health has improved.

If this annex, is the first pages that you're reading, I recommend that you read the rest of the book too. The book contains some pointers for diet and exercise. It also contains some precautions that you take that, I deduct, might save lives. Please read the part about monitoring the heart rate and optimum heart rate. In this annex, I will try to brief some of these points and put them under your view.

I have recommended in the book, that you should buy a small electronic device called heart rate monitor. It consists of a narrow strap for the chest, to observe your heart rate and a watch on your wrist. Please read the part about the optimum heart rate. This number is crucial to know to maximize your exercise level, and to reduce your weight[1], your body fat[1] and improve your health. Some manufacturers have some kind of ringer on the watch that it alarms you, the moment you pass above a setting of your own. If you are in any kind of situation that your heart rate is above the optimum value, then the ring will tell you to stop physical activity, and perhaps sit down or rest. I have heard of stories of old people, who have had a heart attack in the gym or during a simple dancing, simply I deduct, by passing that optimal heart rate too far. Furthermore, for seniors or people with a heart condition, I recommend that ringer could be very useful for exercise and even intimate relations with your spouse.

1: Fit or fat: a book by Dr Covert Bailey

ANNEX SEVEN

THE NECESSARY TO DO LIST TO START THE PROPER EXERCISE

You might have some kind of idea about what you want to use for your exercise. I have a home gym that I put in place of the dining table. My gym consists of a stationary bike, and some weightlifting equipment, specifically some dumbbells. The next is the most important part of the exercise. And that is the heart rate monitor, which is a small electronic device that you can buy from any electronics store or Internet etc. you can see chapter 5 for a lot more explanation on this subject. It is also important especially for joggers, bikers, or people who use stationary bikes. It's good to have a pair of kneepads that you can get from a sports store or the Internet. Some people might choose to get ankle pads, or elbow pads I leave that up to you.

I want to mention that, this book is about improving your health and losing weight. I had no intention to discuss bodybuilding or people who like to exercise with heavy weights.

I recommend, that you invest in yourself. By investing I mean to go to a cardio Specialist. The specialist can determine your optimal heart rate. You will see the importance of this optimal heart rate in the context of the book. I have shown a simple formula recommended by a doctor that will tell you the average person's optimum heart rate. This average is not accurate. In my opinion, the best accurate optimal heart rate can be quoted to you by your cardio specialist.

You need one more specialist, which can be a gym teacher, a trainer, a chiropractor or even an orthopedic specialist. You can choose which one to pick. The importance of this specialist is to tell you, the maximum weight that you can pick up without hurting your back, or your body.

ANNEX EIGHT

HOW TO MAKE YOUR FOOD DELICIOUS WHEN DIETING

In chapter four I brought up the subject of diet foods. In this chapter, I explained that there is a certain amount of protein, carbohydrates, and finally fiber food that is necessary for each meal. In this chapter, I like to explain some ways that I make the food more delicious for my taste.

I think a good breakfast could be several different things. My favorite is milk and cereal with a little bit of honey for sweetness, and some kind of fruit like bananas or strawberries, etc. For lunch and dinner, a good lean type of meat for protein is good. Please refer to chapter 4 for the amounts. In that chapter, other ways are suggested for protein. Then for carbohydrates, a couple of slices of bread or maybe 3 to 4 spoons of cooked rice would suffice. I explained that this diet is all you can eat. When you got the essential parts which are the proteins and carbohydrates, and their amounts right, then you can add all the vegetables that you can eat. That's why your stomach is kind of fooled into believing it is eating a lot of food. Vegetables, specially green vegetables are usually hard to digest, due to fiber in vegetables. Fiber will make the digestion system work harder. And yet none of the green vegetables you eat will stay in the body, and definitely will not be turned into fat. The interesting part is how to make all of these vegetables delicious. A lot of these vegetables taste better when you steam them. Somebody might like to boil them along with the meat and make a stew. I prefer steamed vegetables, along with some delicious sauce. A big part of the delicious diet are spices. You can try different spices and see which one your favorite is. Yogurt can make a very good sauce[1]. Just add a little honey to it, for people who love sweet foods, and some people love to have some hot sauce added, for a spicy taste. They are all kinds of herbs and spices that you can add such as mint or dill weed. And I think cucumber is very good with yogurt. There are a lot of different yogurts. I prefer honey Greek yogurt.

A lot of people love Greek yogurt for example especially if it has honey in it. Let's not forget the ketchup and add vinegar or garlic or all kind of spices to it. You might like the taste of the hot sauce when you add it to the ketchup. Another sauce could be hot sauce and honey. You can add the ketchup or some kind of filler maybe water too. According to the book that I read, garlic powder or garlic as a general rule can help break down the fat in the body and hence make it easier for the body to consume fat. If you are not worried about your social life, then, by all means, add yogurt and garlic powder together with some honey and all kinds of spices for better taste. For example, you can add garlic powder, honey, or herbs to the yogurt. You can add garlic powder, herbs and hot sauce to the ketchup, too. I use about 1/4 of a pound of yogurt for each meal. So make it all you can eat truly, but don't forget the vegetables. Yogurt is known to have the good bacteria and perhaps enzymes to help digestion. Yogurt is known to help lose weight.

HOLD ON YOUR YOUTH LONGER?

In this annex, I will show you the easiest and most effective secret of youth. I have seen and heard the testimonies of the people on TV and books that have revealed this very simple secret of youth. This secret I am talking about, does not include taking any drugs or going through any surgery. No chemicals are necessary. The answer is proper diet and exercise. Read the proper chapters that indicates how to do proper exercise and diet. I have seen a lot of people who do routine exercise and keep a good diet, and they are much older than they look. I also mentioned in the previous chapters that exercise is the best medication that anybody can give themselves. Simply because exercise will keep your body healthy. Healthy body I deduct, would remain younger for longer period of time.

Section 9-1

The following is my speculation: The best way again is, sufficient nutrition for the body. Please see chapter 4 that discusses this issue. The exercise that involves about 30 minutes of rigorous exercise at optimal heart rate, every day is the best in my opinion. At this rate you are most likely to break a sweat. You also get better circulation of blood all over the body. That means good exercise for the kidneys, for the heart and other body organs and surely the muscles of the body. In this book you probably have read the section about using all of your muscles at the same time during an optimal rate exercise. Sweating is very important. The reason is that, sweating gets a lot of bad chemicals out of your body. I believe these bad chemicals that sweat could gets out, are the major contributing factor to fast aging. I also believe that the continuous blood circulation during exercise, could get a lot of bad blood out of the different organs.

This also could be a major factor too. Also exercise makes your body muscles and organs to work hard for the duration of exercise. The more you make your body work and exercise, the more you contribute to your youth.

THE END

www.ingramcontent.com/pod-product-compliance
Lightning Source LLC
Chambersburg PA
CBHW042341030426
42335CB00030B/3427